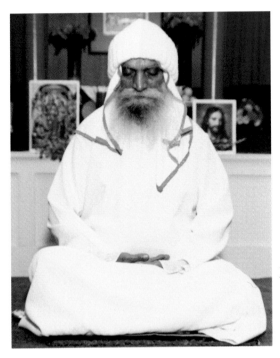

SHRI DHYANYOGI
MADHUSUDANDASJI

(1878–1994)

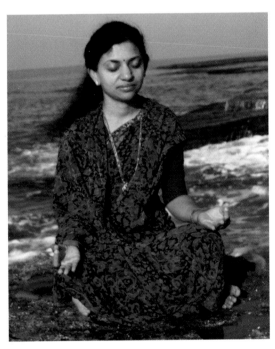

SHRI ANANDI MA

Shakti:
An Introduction to
Kundalini Maha Yoga

SHAKTI

*An Introduction
to Kundalini Maha Yoga*

by

SHRI DHYANYOGI MADHUSUDANDASJI

Published by
Dhyanyoga Centers, Inc.
Antioch, California 94531
First edition 1979
Revised second edition 2000

For inquiries or more information,
please contact Dhyanyoga Centers, Inc. at the addresses below:

Dhyanyoga Centers, Inc.   Shri Anandi Ma Ashram
P.O. Box 3194   Dhyanidham
Antioch, California 94531   AT & P.O. Nikora
or visit our website us at   Dist. BHARUCH
http://www.dyc.org   Gujarat, INDIA

1   3   5   7   9   10   8   6   4   2

Printed in the United States of America.

Library of Congress Cataloging-in-Publication Data Applied For
ISBN 1-883879-08-6 (alk. paper)

Shakti:
An Introduction to
Kundalini Maha Yoga

Books and Recordings
Available from Dhyanyoga Centers

For further information or to place an order,
please visit us on the World Wide Web —
http://www.dyc.org

Note on the Second Edition

This is an expanded edition of the book written by
Shri Dhyanyogi Madhusudandasji in 1979 and published under
the title "*Shakti: Hidden Treasure of Power, Vol. I.*"
Shri Dhyanyogiji left His body in August 1994,
on the anniversary of the birth of Lord Krishna.

The present edition has been expanded to include a talk by
Shri Dhyanyogiji's spiritual heir, Shri Anandi Ma.
This edition is divided into two sections: SECTION I includes
new introductory and biographical material as well as
Shri Anandi Ma's talk entitled "The Kundalini."
SECTION II is composed of original texts
from the first edition by Shri Dhyanyogiji.

Dedication

Gajānanaṁ Namastubhyaṁ Ashṭa Siddhi Pradāyakam |
Duḥkha Dāridyra Hartāraṁ Sarva Vighna Vināśakam || 1 ||

Śrī Rāma Caraṇam Vande Bhaktānugraha Kārakam |
Dīna Bandhurdayā Sindhuḥ Samsārārṇava Tārakam || 2 ||

Dhyātvā Kuṇḍalīnī Śaktiṁ Natvā Tat Pādapankajam |
Smṛitvā Sarasvatiṁ Devīm Idaṁ Grantham Sṛijāmyaham || 3 ||

Iśvaraṁ Gururūpena Hṛidaye Dhārayāmyaham |
Jñānam Ātmā Svarūpasya Dehi Deva Kṛipānidhe || 4 ||

Honor to you, Lord Ganesh, bestower of the eight accomplishments,
destroyer of suffering and poverty, annihilator of all obstacles. (1)

I praise the feet of Sri Rama, who showers kindness on His devotees,
brother to the suffering, the ocean of compassion, the savior from the sea
of birth and death. (2)

Having meditated on Kundalini Shakti, having honored those lotus feet,
having remembered Saraswati Devi, I will write this book. (3)

I will place in my heart the Lord, in the form of the Guru, who gives
knowledge of the true form of the Self, the storehouse of compassion. (4)

෴෴෴

Contents

Section I

Introduction to the Second Edition

Dear Seeker,

I hope and pray that the Divine Energy leads you on the path of truth, bliss and eternal happiness. I feel a great joy to bring forth this second edition of *Shakti*, written by my Guru, Shri Dhyanyogiji.

It is over 20 years since the book was first published in 1979. At that time the science of Kundalini Yoga was largely unknown in the West, thus the readership was limited. But I am sure each book has reached the person who is in sincere quest of the Self. Shri Dhyanyogiji always said, "I believe in quality, not quantity."

When Shri Dhyanyogiji was in the United States, words like Kundalini and Shaktipat were very new to the American public. Much has changed since then, and today these have become familiar terms to persons open to Eastern philosophies and techniques. Substantial growth and benefit have been obtained by hundreds of people. However, there is still a lot to be understood and experienced by thousands more. The Shakti Herself will, of course, pull the right persons toward Her. As is said, when the student is ready, the teacher will appear.

As you hold and read this book, you will surely receive not just the benefit of the written words, but the love and grace of Shri Dhyanyogiji. He will open the doors to realization for you. He may or may not be your teacher, Kundalini Maha Yoga may or may not be your path, yet the grace of Ma Kundalini Shakti and the grace of a saint, through the *Guru Tattva*, will always be yours. So, fear not, have faith, work hard and the goal is sure to be reached. I hope I can see you personally at a meditation somewhere, and my love and blessings are always with you. Love and blessings pour out from the depth of my heart for you to realize your Self. Seek and you shall receive.

September 2000
Antioch, California
Shri Anandi Ma

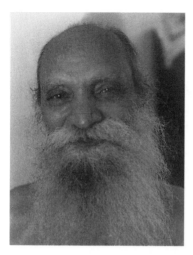

Shri Dhyanyogi Madhusudandasji

The Teachers of the Lineage

"I have come here for the dissemination of spiritual knowledge. My message is straightforward; I invite you all to come, sit, meditate, experience and judge for yourself. May God bless you all."

SHRI DHYANYOGI MADHUSUDANDAS-JI (1878–1994) was a great saint, whose search for spiritual enlightenment took place during another era, in an India that no longer exists. He walked barefoot across India, in the 1890's and early 1900's, through what were then jungles, but are now cleared and settled lands, meeting saints living in seclusion, completely detached from the mundane world.

Born in the small village of Durgadih in Bihar state, India, Shri Dhyanyogi-ji* was a very spiritual child. Before His birth, His mother had a vision of Lord Krishna, indicating the coming of a great being. His spiritual quest began in earnest at age 7 when He left home in search of God. Although He was quickly found by His parents, He left home again for good at age 13. The next 30 years were spent traveling all over India learning whatever the saints and yogis would teach Him.

---

* The suffix "ji" added to a name denotes respect.

He mastered Mantra, Yantra, Hatha, Raja and Jnana Yogas, and became adept at yogic philosophies and scriptures. Yet after 30 years of austerities and intense searching, He still had not attained His highest goal, the ultimate encounter with God. Finally, in 1921 on Mt. Abu, He came into the presence of His final teacher, a great master named Shri Yogiraj Parameshwardasji, who gave Him Shaktipat initiation. He immediately went into the highest state of *samadhi*, attained the ultimate goal of God realization, and remained in that condition for three days.

Shri Dhyanyogiji was a unique being. As a result of His own search, and, through the grace and guidance of Shri Parameshwardasji, He became a master of Kundalini Maha Yoga, with the power to awaken the dormant Kundalini in spiritual aspirants.

He founded a small ashram in the village of Bandhwad, in Gujarat state, India, where He carried on His work and teachings. In 1960, He was inspired to begin public instruction in Kundalini Maha Yoga and to conduct group meditation programs throughout India. In doing so, Shri Dhyanyogiji became the first teacher in the entire history of this multi-thousand-year lineage to come out into the open and work at a mass level to raise humanity's consciousness.

He came to America in 1976 as part of His worldwide mission to help spiritual seekers. During His four years here, He established local groups from coast to coast and initiated thousands into the path of Kundalini Maha Yoga. He returned to India in 1980 and spent His remaining years in residence in Ahmedabad, in Gujarat state. To His students' great sorrow, Shri Dhyanyogiji consciously left His physical body after 116 years, entering *Mahasamadhi* on August 29, 1994, the anniversary of Lord Krishna's birth.

Shri Dhyanyogiji's simple, pure love, and devotion to the welfare of mankind, changed the hearts of the thousands of people whose lives He touched. Today, His energy continues to work at the subtle level and through His spiritual heir, Shri Anandi Ma.

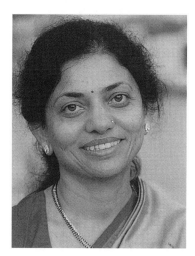

Shri Anandi Ma

SHRI ANANDI MA is Shri Dhyanyogiji's spiritual heir and was known for many years as Asha Ma or Ashadevi. In January 1993, Shri Dhyanyogiji gave Her the spiritual name Anandi Ma, which means "One who is in Bliss and keeps others in Bliss." Her early years passed in a quiet and uneventful manner, in an environment rich with spiritual practice and energy. One day in 1972, at the age of 14, She spontaneously entered a very deep, meditative state. In Her own words, She saw "the light of a million suns," and in the same moment had a vision of the Divine Mother, and merged with Her. Following this experience Shri Anandi Ma was constantly going into meditative states. Her father went to Shri Dhyanyogiji and asked Him to come meet Her, and provide guidance and assistance. Shri Dhyanyogiji went to their home and woke Her from a deep meditative state. Later that day He asked Her to describe Her vision of the Divine Mother. "Did you see Her as a picture, a statue, a living being?" Shri Anandi Ma answered, "Just as I see you now." That same day, Shri Dhyanyogiji said Shri Anandi Ma was the most spiritually advanced person, for Her age, He had ever met. With

Her parents' consent, She left home shortly after receiving Shaktipat to stay permanently with Shri Dhyanyogiji.

He took Her under His wing and trained Her to control and radiate Her energies for the welfare of humanity, especially by giving Shaktipat. He said, "I have been asked by my Guru to hand over the powers of this lineage to Her," and put aside all His major activities to work almost exclusively with Her, day and night, for four years. During this period Shri Anandi Ma would enter profound states of meditation for hours or days at a time. From the beginning, Shri Anandi Ma worked alongside Shri Dhyanyogiji wherever He traveled, and accompanied Him when He came to America in 1976.

When Shri Dhyanyogiji returned to India in 1980, He told Shri Anandi Ma and Shri Dileepji to marry and continue His work together. Shri Dileepji, like Shri Anandi Ma, has been Shri Dhyanyogiji's student since his early teens, accompanying Him in His travels. With Shri Dhyanyogiji's guidance and blessings, Shri Dileepji performed intense spiritual practices, mastered many yogic disciplines, and became one of His most advanced disciples. Shri Dileepji is empowered by Shri Dhyanyogiji to perform Shaktipat initiation.

Today, Shri Anandi Ma and Shri Dileepji travel extensively in India, the United States and Europe, conducting meditation programs and yoga retreats. They provide spiritual guidance and Shaktipat initiation to sincere seekers. As part of Her role as Shri Dhyanyogiji's spiritual heir, Shri Anandi Ma has also assumed the responsibility for continuing the humanitarian works begun during Shri Dhyanyogiji's lifetime. These include operating a hospital, sponsoring eye surgery camps, and providing food for the poor. In all these works, She continues to spread the love and light of Her lineage and of Her beloved *sadguru*, Shri Dhyanyogi Madhusudandasji.

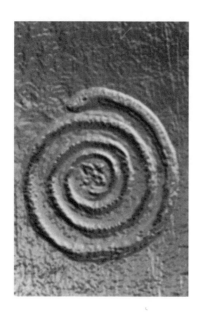

The Kundalini

*Originally presented as a discourse
by Shri Anandi Ma at a
public meditation program held
in Woodbury, Connecticut
in October 1998.*

Paraashakti Kundalini Vishatantu Taniyasi

"She is the Supreme Energy, as fine as the filament of the lotus stalk."

Shaktihi Kundaliniti Vishwajanani Vyapaara Vadhodhyamaa

"She is the Power known as Kundalini, engaged in the work of creating the universe."

Muladhaare Mulavidyaam Vidyutkoti Samaaprabaam
Suryakoti Pratikaasham Chandrakoti Tuvaampriye

"She is the root of all knowledge, having the brilliance of millions of lightnings and millions of suns put together.

At the same time, She is cool and pleasing like the energy of millions of moons together."

Lalita Sahasranama

DEAR BROTHERS AND SISTERS, since the very beginning of Creation, with the manifestation of the individual soul in the human body, the search for eternal and complete bliss has been constant. In order to acquire this inner state, to achieve the Absolute Truth, many beings all across the world, including many in India, have dedicated their lives to the search for different means to achieve that end. As a result, over the centuries, different paths with different techniques have become available to reach this inner state.

Over the centuries many of these techniques and paths became known externally, and some were taught quite freely. But often paths were kept hidden. Some were kept secret because they involved more serious efforts, and the outcomes were rather strong as well. Thus they required a greater level of inner discipline. At times these paths manifested inner faculties and powers that teachers felt might be misused. So in order to prevent such misuse, they were kept well hidden, imparted selectively only to qualified persons.

For thousands of years, this particular path of Kundalini Maha Yoga was kept rather secret. It is only over the past 30 or 40 years that a few teachers have come out in the open and made these priceless teachings available to the general public for their welfare.

It is a very natural process, yet even to this day, many consider it quite mysterious. But it is only a lack of knowledge or understanding that creates the idea of something being strange or mysterious.

Today we have instrumentation that can predict the weather; we know when events like earthquakes are likely to occur. We can know all this, yet there seems to be no power to stop these events. However, even in these days, there are beings, yogis, who do have the capacity to stop such events from occurring in creation. For the most part, they will not use their energies to bring about such modifications, but rather follow the laws of creation and of nature. By and large, following their intuition, they allow things to unfold as they are destined to be. In rare instances, however, they may use their energies in this way to help protect humanity.

Over the years, many of us had several such experiences with Shri Dhyanyogiji. Often when it was raining, He would simply look up into the sky and it would stop; all of a sudden the weather would change. And when rain was needed, particularly in areas and times of drought in India, He would simply go to the areas, look up at the sky, and shortly thereafter there would be a downpour. This, of course, is not the goal or the aim of the path, but it does indicate that the ability to understand and control these outer forces can occur when one has understood oneself completely and can control the inner energies, particularly the Kundalini.

It is important to try and understand what the Kundalini is.

The Indian scriptures describe it endlessly. In the *Lalita Sahasranama*, for example, it is said that it is the most subtle energy, more subtle than the finest filament of a lotus stalk. It is known as Parashakti or Adishakti, the Prime Energy, the first energy, the energy which is beyond all energies, the energy which was before manifestation of creation, caused creation itself, and will still remain constant after creation is dissolved.

The yogis, based upon their inner experiences, have described the Kundalini in many ways. For example, they say it is that energy which contains within itself the light, the brilliance, and the heat of thousands of suns put together. It is that energy which combines thousands of lightning bolts together. It is that energy which has the coolness and the luminosity of thousands of moons simultaneously. It is all this in one energy, and much more.

The yogis in more recent times have described it as that energy which is a sum total of all the electrical energy that has been produced up to this moment and that will be produced as long as this creation exists. So all that energy put together is the Kundalini energy. Yet, as the yogis say, it is even beyond all these descriptions.

The most important thing is the inner experience that first has to be had with and from the energy within. The goal of this energy is to attain realization, to take you back to the cause from which we have all come.

This is the direct experience of the yogis over thousands of years. For that matter, all the Indian scriptures have come from direct experience. They do not come from the intellect, but from things that yogis experienced, then met and discussed. And when they found that they had received identical experiences, and when those were definitely known to be free of the limitations of the human mind, intelligence and ego, then and then only were they declared a scripture. So basically, these sciences do not come from the intellect but from the purely spiritual level.

The human mind, although extremely powerful, can be extremely limiting. Even in giving this talk, the mind of the teacher becomes restricted in order to present experiential knowledge via the intellect. And each listener's own level of intelligence and mind will process it differently. Certainly, if you were all asked to write down what has just been said, you would all come up with different things.

The Kundalini is divided into two aspects. One, again, is the Universal Energy, which is unmanifested, yet still brings about all of the functions in external creation. And then within the body of each individual that same energy has manifested as the personal Kundalini. The yogis visualized this energy in a coiled state at the base of the human spine. The Sanskrit term for a coil is *kundal*, and that's why they call it the Kundalini.

But it must be understood that universally the energy is identical, one and the same, for all humanity. There is no difference. It may be named differently, but the inner experience at the higher level is identical for one and all.

It is the Kundalini that, in fact, starts the creation of the human body in the fetus. The first part of the creation, at the physical level, is the brain. At the subtle level, the chakras are formed, the first being the *Sahasrar* at the top of the head, which is the most important center in the body. The brain is indeed the control center of the human body, at the physical level. At the subtle level, all the subtle functions, and what are known as the *nadis* — the subtle energy pathways — are controlled by the sahasrar chakra.

One of the Kundalini's most important functions at the human level is the mind. The seat of the human mind is said to be in what is known as the *manas* chakra, which is at the third eye center. As we know, all the senses are controlled by the brain, and at the subtle level, by the sahasrar chakra. All of these are within the head and face area — the eyes, the ears, the nose, the tongue — the senses of seeing, hearing, smelling, tasting — these are all governed at the subtle level through the sahasrar chakra at the top of the head.

All the critical and vital functions are controlled by the brain at the physical level, but the brain is deriving its energy from something very subtle, and that is the sahasrar chakra. When we want to think deeply or concentrate, we may close our eyes and place our hands on our head. We don't place them on the heart or the leg. When we want to remember something, or when we make a stupid mistake, we may bang our head and say, "Oh, how stupid I am." These automatic actions reflect the subtle functioning of the energy in this area.

For those who are initiated and are practicing, or connected to a teacher and a lineage, the sahasrar chakra becomes the seat of the Guru within each disciple, particularly after the teacher leaves the physical world. So for disciples, a lot of concentration is to be done at the sahasrar chakra.

When the physical body is being formed, it is the *prana* energy, which is a radiation or an extension of the soul, which comes first and begins the formation. Then the Kundalini enters, and this is the main aspect of the soul. It is between the fifth and the sixth month that the soul is said to really enter the body. Prior to that, the preparation to hold that energy takes place so that the soul can truly enter. Finally comes the time for the soul to enter. It is said to take birth based upon its *samskaras* (past mind impressions). And it takes whatever karma it wants to enjoy or suffer in that lifetime from the storehouse of its actions of several lifetimes. The soul then enters the body with its faults and with its energies, and with what we call genetic predispositions. But actually it is the soul which has predetermined, very, very precisely, exactly what illnesses and dispositions it is going to inherit.

It is similar to when you build a home. You may purchase a lot and start the construction, but until the house is ready you do not move in. You may visit the site, however, directing things as per your wishes. Similarly, several months before the soul enters the body, it will generally hover around the would-be mother, preparing to enter the body.

It is the Kundalini energy that is primarily responsible for creating the body. It begins with the subtleties. First the sahasrar chakra is formed, then it descends along the path of the spinal column, and the spinal column is formed physically as well. Then within, at the subtle level, the different energy centers — the chakras — are formed. Then internal organs and the rest of the body are finally formed.

So, again, at the fifth month, the body is more or less formed so that it can hold the energy of the soul. It is then that the soul descends into the body. The growth continues until the ninth month, when birth occurs. The soul finally enters, with what is known as the prana or the *chi*, as most of you might know it. Then the other aspects begin to take hold — the mind, the intellect, and the ego — and then the five organs of action — *karmendriya* — and the five senses of knowledge — *jnanendriya*.

The Kundalini energy then goes to the base of the spine and becomes dormant. Yet even though it is dormant, it is still supporting the physical body and, at a subtle level, keeping everything functioning.

When the child is born, he or she may continue to evolve, as we understand it, in an external way. But, as the yogis say, that person is actually going through three levels of experiences through the three states of consciousness — that is the state of being awake, the state of sleeping, and the state of dreaming. The fourth state, *turiya*, which transcends the other three, is the state of absolute knowledge and is experienced only by the yogis. This state can be experienced only after the Kundalini is awakened.

The yogis have found that when the consciousness is at the sahasrar chakra, and thus the soul is aware of its absolute state, at that time it is constantly repeating a mantra. This mantra is known as "*Soham*," which means that "You and I are one;" as Christ said, "I and my father are one." That is the absolute awareness of the consciousness of the soul at that time, which the yogis experience in their deepest states of meditation. And when the soul is in the womb, when the awareness is still not very external or physical, it is aware of the consciousness that "You and I are one."

As the child is born, however, the consciousness begins to descend. There are what are known as *bija* letters or mantras on all of the chakras; when the soul descends to the heart area it associates with that reality, and the first letter of the chakra there is "ka." So instead of "Soham" the soul begins to be restricted to the experience of "*Koham*," which means "Who am I?". Thus awareness has been lost.

And finally, the consciousness descends to be with the Kundalini at the base of the spine, to the first chakra, known as the *muladhara* ("*mul*" is root; "*adhar*" is support). That is where the Kundalini resides, and when the consciousness has descended to the base of the spine, then the awareness that remains is "*Dehoham*," which means "I am the body." To make matters worse, everything vibrating around us enforces that impression. If you ask your parents who you are, they will say, "You are my son," "You are my daughter," "This is your name." And then friends, relatives, everyone around us, and all the material factors reinforce that fact over and over and over again, that you are nothing except the body.

At that point the soul is said to be completely individualized, it is what we call a "conditioned soul." Although it is absolute, because of external factors and limitations that the individual creates through the mind, intellect and ego, it becomes very, very physical, in a sense. And then, as long as the Kundalini remains dormant at the base of the spine, that level of consciousness remains.

The Kundalini rests with its head downward. But if through some means it is activated, it turns around and faces upward. Once that happens, consciousness begins to change. The person then at least begins to ask the question, "Who am I?"

Finally, through further practices, the Kundalini has to be brought back to the top of the head. When it reaches the sahasrar again, then all restrictions that keep it bound to the physical and material level drop away, and the final realization of "You and I are one" manifests for the individual. So "Soham" again becomes the awareness.

That is the key to spiritual evolution. When the force is downward, you are bound, you are restricted, you are human; but when the force is reversed, then, as the scriptures say, you are no longer human; you are then God.

For thousands of years, as the yogis researched, they found that no matter what one practiced, no matter what one believed, the key to evolution was the awakening and activation of this energy. Again, what it is called is secondary, but this inner force needs to be active through whatever techniques, through whatever belief systems one has adopted. And so this energy became a key factor for the yogis to explore.

Of course, there are many ways in which the Kundalini energy can be awakened, but the simplest and most direct is the process of shaktipat. Shaktipat means the transmission or the giving of energy. Those yogis who have achieved complete control and mastery over their own vital force — the prana — can transmit this energy to others. They may do it simply by touching another person. They may do it by their will power — *sankalpa* — sometimes over thousands of miles. Yogis are known to transmit energy simply by gazing at a person, transmitting energy through their eyes. And lastly, sound is used to give energy; in India, mantras in particular are used.

Once the Kundalini is awakened, all the person needs to do is practice, to meditate regularly; and one can adopt whatever other support for the practices one may like. But again, the key is through the practice to raise the energy, slowly but surely, along the spine, to open up the chakras, and finally bring it to the crown chakra. Then the conditioned soul no longer remains conditioned but becomes the Absolute.

As the Kundalini unfolds with regular practice, besides fulfilling the most important goal of life, which is self-realization, it manifests other benefits in day-to-day living. These include the enhancement of overall physical strength and energy, and keeping the body fit and immune to illnesses. A lot of healing is also known to occur spontaneously. The energy enhances the mental and intellectual faculties. But most of all it brings inner peace and balance; and these are the most important factors for happiness while we are still in the physical body.

This is a universal science of spiritual growth, and the most important thing is the direct, personal, inner experience. If you want to understand what sweetness is, you have to eat some sugar, something sweet. No one can describe that for you. Therefore, in reality, nothing has to be said, because everything only needs to be experienced. As Dhyanyogiji simply said, "Come, sit, meditate, and experience."

To conclude, I would like to shower my love and blessings upon you. May you all reach the goal of life, and as you reach it, may the days ahead be filled with the grace of the divine. May you be free from all obstacles, and may inner peace, joy, and happiness always be with you.

Sarve Bhavantu Sukhinah	May everyone everywhere be happy
Sarve Santu Niramayah	Let each and every heart be filled with love, peace, and joy
Sarve Bhadrani Pashyantu	May all miseries be destroyed
Ma Kaschid Dukhabhag Bhavet	
Ma Kaschid Dukhabhag Bhavet	And may each and every soul thirst to reach God
Om shantih shantih shantih	Om, peace, peace, peace

16

Section II

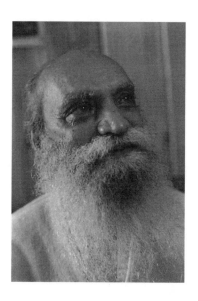

Introduction from the First Edition

by Shri Dhyanyogi Madhusudandasji

FOR THE PAST SEVERAL DECADES, YOGA, a spiritual discipline from India, has been a subject of interest to people of this country. Consequently, I believe that many of you are already familiar with its terminology. The purpose of this Introduction is to acquaint you with the Shakti, or Kundalini, and the related form of yoga known as Kundalini Maha Yoga.

The principle on which it is based is very simple. In every human being there is a source of divine energy, called Kundalini in Sanskrit. It exists within the individual in two states, one dormant and one awakened and active. When it is dormant, a person leads an unhappy, unfulfilled life. The understanding of the universe is restricted and everything is perceived and interpreted according to a limited capacity. When the Kundalini is aroused and active, a person makes rapid progress on the path of spiritual evolution. The full potential of body and mind are realized, inner peace, harmony and integration are attained, and ultimately the sublime truth of unity in diversity is experienced — the fact that all life is one seamless fabric.

The purpose of this yoga is to awaken the Kundalini if it is dormant and to intensify its activity if it has been aroused. Thus, Kundalini Maha Yoga is a direct method of spiritual evolution, and as such its importance is obvious. There are also side benefits, such as the spontaneous healing of many diseases of body and mind.

A powerful yogi can awaken the Kundalini by a transfer of his or her energy to the student; this acts as the initial impetus. The process is called Shaktipat *(Shakti* meaning "power" or "energy" in Sanskrit, and *pata* meaning "transfer.") Through the grace and advice of my own guru, who gave me Shaktipat many years ago in India, I have been able to do Shaktipat on thousands of people both here and abroad. Because of this experience, I have been encouraged to bring Kundalini Maha Yoga to your attention so that it may aid the spiritual endeavors of people in America.

First, let us look at the role Kundalini Maha Yoga can play in solving the problems of the world. As we all know, during the past several decades scientific development has taken place at a staggering rate. It is both a joy and a surprise to watch science progress. However, since the storehouse of nature is limitless, the more we know, the more remains to be known. It is obvious that no one person can understand nature fully. Thus, there is a clear need to further develop the powers of the intellect, the capacity to comprehend, and also to develop the general powers of the mind to the extent that faculties as yet unused may be involved.

In addition, the need for sound mental health cannot be overlooked. Much remains to be accomplished in the area of both mental and physical health. Many serious diseases still threaten mankind and neurotic and psychotic behavior abounds. But a strong body and mind are not sufficient. Today, despite our many developments, there is much fear, hatred and disharmony between individuals, communities and nations. This has led to the buildup of destructive weapons and the grave possibility of thermonuclear war. Peace, though much desired, has not been attained.

A basic cause of these problems is that the general level of conscience, consciousness and other spiritual qualities has not evolved to the same extent that the material side of civilization has. We are in a state of unbalanced development, lacking on the spiritual side. Therefore, to attain what is missing — peace, harmony and unity with all beings — it is necessary to realize that the entire universe is the creation of God, that all life is one and that we all are one. This realization is spiritual realization, not the merely intellectual comprehension of an ideal. Spiritual evolution alone is the solution to the problems facing us. Kundalini Maha Yoga is a way to spiritual evolution and therefore a significant tool for the development of mankind on the spiritual plane. It is a path to peace, prosperity, unity and love.

In this book, I will describe in some detail the yogic theory of the Kundalini. In brief outline, the Kundalini is divine energy which manifests in both cosmic and personal form. The cosmic form is the entire universe, the entire interconnected pattern of all that is and becomes. The personal form is the pattern of that energy within each individual living being.

Yogis believe that the development of the universe is cyclic. Each cycle consists of creation, maintenance and destruction, just as each life does on a smaller scale. When a cycle of the universe is completed, all individuals attain liberation in the general dissolution of all limiting forms. But the individual does not have to await the end of the cycle for his liberation. With the awakening of the Kundalini, he may attain it in one lifetime.

In my own training period of over 30 years, I had contacts with large numbers of capable yogis. I did severe austerities at places of exceptional spiritual energy; Chitrakut, Girnar, the Himalayas and on Mt. Abu. Then, by the grace of God, I met my Guru who performed Shaktipat on me. Since that time, I have done Shaktipat on a large number of people, thus awakening their Kundalini, which has brought them good health and peace of mind, and has led them along the spiritual path.

I have come for the dissemination of spiritual knowledge. It is my hope that this book will aid this purpose. I wish to express my thanks to all the people who helped in preparing this book. I consider the whole world to be my family. My message is straightforward. I invite you all to come, sit, meditate, experience and judge for yourselves. May God bless you all.

February 1979
Los Angeles, California
Shri Dhyanyogi Madhusudandasji

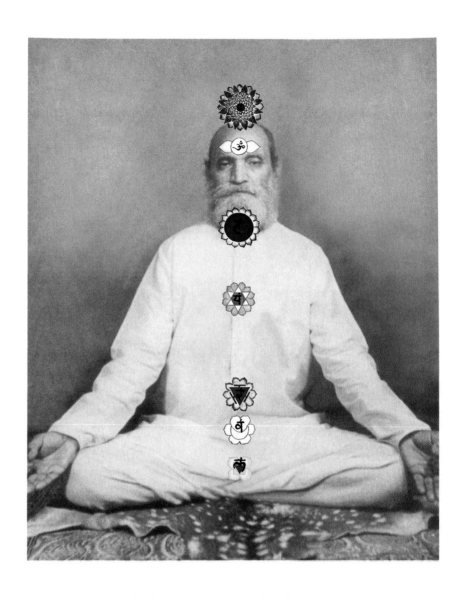

"This gross physical substance
comes into being
from the subtle."

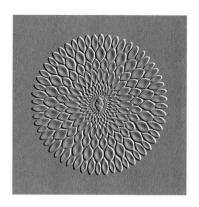

What is Kundalini?

by Shri Dhyanyogi Madhusudandasji

YOGIS SAY THAT THERE ARE MANY similarities between the human body and the entire universe, the microcosm and the macrocosm. The Upanishads say that in the region of the heart is a hollow space the size of the tip of the thumb that contains all things. All elements, all things, regardless of whether they are present or absent in the immediate external environment, are present in this microcosmic universe in the heart.

There are 101 types of nadis, the channels through which prana flows in the subtle body. One called *Hita* is of particular significance here, for just as a road connects two towns, this nadi is connected to the Sun and energy is collected from the Sun through it. By concentrating on this nadi, one can achieve various kinds of powers, like seeing things happening very far away, having the ability to do healing, having visions of gods, saints or previous incarnations.

In this world, on both the subtle and the physical level, although the atoms and molecules are in constant motion through their mutual attraction and repulsion, many of the laws of their behavior are unknown. Consider, on the physical level, the planet Earth. Her dimensions and composition are well known. She has a surface of 512 million square kilometers. The Sun is vastly larger and is over 90 million miles away from the Earth. The star called Jyestha in Indian astronomy is many times greater than the Sun and other stars are known to be even larger. The number of stars within this galaxy cannot be counted and there are innumerable galaxies within that part of the universe that our telescopes can reach and many, many solar systems within each of them. The nearest star is so far away that its light takes more than four years to reach the Earth.

Yogis believe that life exists around millions of stars, based on the searches made up to this time. Great sages have described the universe as endless. One begins to lose one's mind when the extent of this universal creation is considered. Such is the physical universe.

This gross physical substance comes into being from the subtle. The atomic structure of the elements of nature is also full of wonders. Every substance in this world is composed of molecules and atoms with their fields of moving charged particles. It has been found that the general laws of the substantial world hold true in many ways for the subatomic world also. Ongoing research is constantly revising and perfecting its understanding. It cannot be said that we know all that there is to know. Initially, it was thought that the atom was indivisible—that is what its very name means—but today it has been broken up and the analysis of its many parts is continuing. Various types of research are being done in this area. Weapons, which could destroy the entire world in a moment, have been invented using this knowledge. Even the researchers become uneasy when they consider the destructive power of these weapons. Research is also being done on constructive uses for these energies. I hope they will be successful.

The axis through the North and South Poles maintains the balance of the Earth. The Earth rotates around this axis and revolves about the Sun in a fixed orbit because of the physical forces operating around these poles. Some scientists believe that the Earth would be thrown many millions of miles off its present orbit if there were major changes at the poles, so it is considered unwise to conduct heavy experiments near them. Similarly, in the human body, the Sahasrara chakra in the crown of the head and the Muladhara chakra at the base of the spinal column are the poles of the energy system, the two main centers of the body. All energies, all powers and all experiences are stored between these two centers.

We know the major planets of our solar system: the Moon, Mercury, Venus, Mars, Jupiter, Saturn, Uranus, Neptune, Pluto and so forth. But everything is not known. In the course of time, many new things are likely to be found. That is the nature of the universe.

Now let us talk more about the human body. It is made up of natural elements like all bodies but has capacities not found in other animals. Man has superior intelligence, discretion and thinking abilities and has the art of writing and other faculties no other animal known to us has.

By using the human body as a vehicle and by exerting oneself in the right direction, one can see God and finally become one with Him. Meditating on the subtle structure of the body leads to that end. That is why the scriptures say: Fire is in the form of speech in the mouth, the wind is in the form of energy in the nose, the Sun with the power of sight is in the eyes, the directions of space as sound is in the ears, *vayu* as protection against disease is in the skin, the Moon is in the form of the mind in the heart, death is in the form of *apana-vayu* in the navel, and water is in the form of semen in the senses of enjoyment.

According to Indian Astrology, the essence of the Sun is in the form of the soul, the Moon in the form of the mind, Mars in the form of blood, Mercury in the form of speech, Jupiter in the form of knowledge, Venus in the form of seminal fluid, and Saturn is the agent of the experiences of joy and misery in the body.

Expansion and contraction, attraction and repulsion are movements constantly going on in the universe. After finishing a course of development, creation returns to its original condition. After a time, a kind of repeated tremor begins and the energy of God in the form of Kundalini Shakti, by creating vibrations, brings about a new creation in eight archetypal forms: solid, liquid, gaseous, radiant, energy, space, consciousness, intelligence and ego. In the *Bhagavad Gita* it is said:

> "Earth, water, fire, wind, space, consciousness, intellect and ego: thus my Prakriti has been divided into eight parts."
>
> (*Bhagavad Gita*, Chap. 7, Verse 4)

Creation begins with the union of *Purusha* and *Prakriti*, that is, by the union of God and Maya Shakti. God creates this universe from Himself by producing subtle energies by a process akin to autosuggestion. This is like the generation of sparks from a fire. The individual manifestation of the Kundalini is like a spark from the cosmic Kundalini. This personal form of Kundalini is responsible for the creation of an individual.

After the *jiva*, the individualized focus of consciousness, separates from God, it acquires certain attributes including the senses and a feeling of ego. At first it is very pure and full of knowledge, but as it comes under the full spell of Maya it becomes like a caged animal.

> "My eternal part, having become a living being in the world of life, commands the indriyas (the organs of sense and action) with the mind as the sixth (sense), fixed in Prakriti (Nature)." [7]

> "When the Atma obtains a body and also when he leaves one, he takes these (indriyas and mind) and goes, like the wind takes scents from their sources." [8]

> "Inhabiting the organs of hearing, sight, touch, taste, smell and thought, He enjoys the objects of the senses." [9]

> "The deluded do not discover Him united with the gunas (the qualities of Nature), who departs or stays or enjoys. But they who have the eye of knowledge see (Him)." [10]

> *(Bhagavad Gita,* Chap. 15, verses 7–10)

Many forms of energy are circular in nature. If you fly in a straight line over the surface of the Earth long enough, you will come back to where you started. Nature proceeds by expansion and contraction. Since time immemorial, these forces of creation and destruction have operated in a circular manner.

Chakra Positions

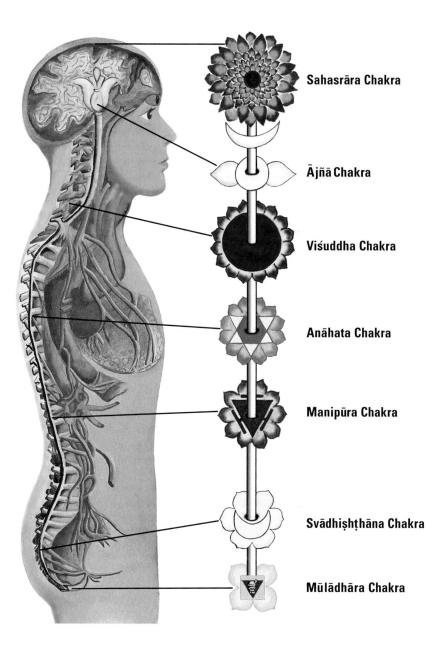

Sahasrāra Chakra

Ājñā Chakra

Viśuddha Chakra

Anāhata Chakra

Manipūra Chakra

Svādhiṣṭhāna Chakra

Mūlādhāra Chakra

*To gain knowledge of the chakras, the mantra So'Ham-Hansaḥ
should be recited during the 21,600 breaths taken daily.
Each chakra requires a specific number of repetitions.*

Sahasrara Chakra

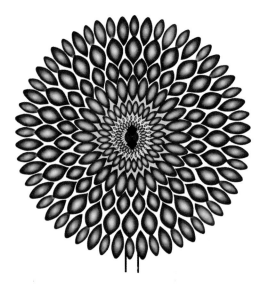

Location	Brain (at Crown of Head)
Number of Petals	One thousand
Color	Red
Prana-Vayu	Vyana
Presiding Deity	Paramatma
Quality	Sattva
Seed Letter	Visarga :
Results of Meditation	Liberation
So'Ham Hansaha Repetitions	One thousand

WHEN A CHILD IS CREATED through the union of male and female energies in a mother's womb, Shakti first forms the Sahasrara in the head. Many forces are stored there. The Sahasrara has a thousand petals and is red in color. Its presiding deity is Paramatma. The prana-vayu, vital air energy, named vyana operates there, and the quality of the Shakti there is *sattvic*. Its seed letter is the *visarga*. Meditation on this chakra brings liberation.

After forming the Sahasrara chakra in the brain, the Kundalini Shakti forms the spinal column from the nerves that branch from the brain. Just as currents are created in the flow of a river, so the energy forms six centers, called chakras, in the flow pattern through the spinal column.

In the *Yoga Sutra* of Patanjali Muni, it is said:

> "In the light from the head, you can see the siddhas and other deities."

> [III-33]

Ajna Chakra

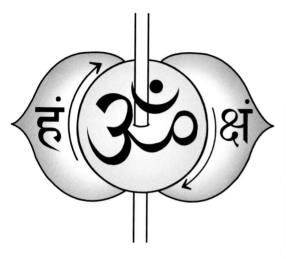

Location	Between eyebrows
Number of Petals	Two
Color	White
Shape	Round
Related Element	Manas-Tattva
Prana-Vayu	Prana
Presiding Deity	Jivatma
Quality	Pure Sattva
Seed Letter	Aum
Results of Meditation	Nectar Unlimited vision Control of adverse circumstances
***So'Ham Hansaha* Repetitions**	One thousand

KUNDALINI NEXT FORMS THE AJNA CHAKRA between the eyebrows. It is round in shape and has two white petals. Its related element is the manas-tattva, mind element, and its prana-vayu is prana. The presiding deity is Atma and its quality is pure sattva. The bija mantra or seed letter is Aum. Meditation on this chakra brings nectar, unlimited vision and control over adverse circumstances.

A student becomes more powerful in all respects by meditating on this chakra. When it is fully opened, one can see anywhere, into every place and time, without limitation. If one desires to do so, one can control adverse circumstances. That is why it is called the Ajna (towards knowledge) chakra. In the upward movement of the Kundalini during meditation, after crossing this chakra, the Shakti can enter the Sahasrara without any further problems. That stage is called the union of the jiva, the individualized being, with God.

Vishuddha Chakra

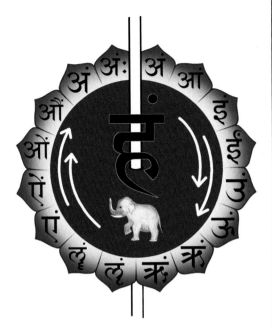

Location	Base of throat
Number of Petals	Sixteen
Color	Dark Blue
Shape	Round
Related Element	Space
Prana-Vayu	Udana
Presiding Deity	Jivatma
Quality	Sattva
Seed Letter	Ham हं
Vehicle of Kundalini	Elephant
Results of Meditation	Purification of mental attitude and physical body Knowledge Intense joy
So'Ham Hansaha Repetitions	One thousand

AFTER FORMING THE AJNA CHAKRA, the Kundalini forms the Vishuddha chakra in the throat region. It has sixteen dark blue petals and is round in shape. It is related to the element *akasha* (space or sky) and its prana-vayu is udana. The presiding deity is Jivatma and the quality sattva. The seed letter is Ham. The vehicle of the Kundalini at this chakra is the elephant. Meditation on this chakra brings a purification of mental attitudes and the attainment of siddhis. One is showered with knowledge and experiences intense joy. The physical body is also purified and diseases, impurities and physical difficulties are eliminated. That is why this chakra is called Vishuddha (completely cleansed).

Patanjali Muni says:

> "In the cavity of the throat, hunger and thirst are turned away."
>
> [*Yoga Sutra*, III-31]

> "From the conquest of the udana, water, mud, thorns, etc., become harmless; and one can die at will."
>
> [Ibid. III-40]

Anahata Chakra

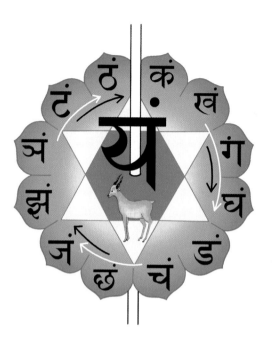

Location	Heart
Number of Petals	Twelve
Color	Green
Shape	Hexagon (formed by six-pointed star)
Related Element	Air
Prana-Vayu	Prana
Presiding Deity	Maheshvara
Quality	Sattva with some rajas
Seed Letter	Yam यं
Vehicle of Kundalini	Antelope
Results of Meditation	Material gains Knowledge
So'Ham Hansaha Repetitions	Six thousand

THE KUNDALINI SHAKTI NEXT FORMS THE ANAHATA CHAKRA in the region of the heart. It has twelve green petals and a hexagon shape. It is related to the element air, and its prana-vayu is prana. The presiding deity is Maheshvara and although its quality is still sattva, that quality is no longer pure as it was in the Ajna chakra but is now mixed with *rajas*. The seed letter is Yam and the vehicle is an antelope. Continuous sounds exist in this chakra including the sounds of Brahma and Aum. These are the first sounds created during the formation of the universe and their location in this chakra means that it is created spontaneously as soon as the Shakti is present. Anahata means unbeaten or unwounded and refers to the Aum sound that is not produced by percussion. The name also suggests the pristine quality of undyed (i.e. unwounded) new cloth. Various types of material benefits and knowledge come from concentration on this chakra.

Patanjali Muni mentions one:

> "In the heart is understanding of the mind. "
>
> [*Yoga Sutra*, III-35]

31

Manipura Chakra

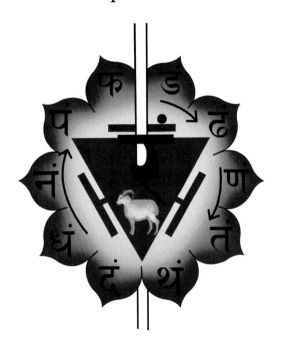

Location	Navel
Number of Petals	Ten
Color	Red
Shape	Triangle
Related Element	Fire
Prana-Vayu	Samana
Presiding Deity	Vishnu
Quality	Rajas
Seed Letter	Ram रं
Vehicle of Kundalini	The Ram
Results of Meditation	Knowledge of internal function of physical body
So'Ham Hansaha Repetitions	Six thousand

DESCENDING FURTHER, the Kundalini creates the fifth or Manipura chakra. It is located at the navel, has ten red petals and a triangle shape. Its element is fire (radiant energy). The prana-vayu is samana, the deity Vishnu, the quality rajas, the seed letter Ram and the vehicle a ram. This chakra is the center of the human body and all of the main nadis meet there. It is very important to the functioning of the body. A child in the womb is connected to the mother through the umbilical cord attached near this center and is fed from there only.

Yogis believe that during times of astral travel, the subtle body and the physical body remain attached to each other by a subtle cord coming out through this center. Just as a high flying kite is drawn back by its connecting string after traveling great distances, so the subtle body is pulled back to the center of the physical body by this cord. The cord is silvery and shining like a jewel (*mani*), and the chakra is its city (*pura*) or home, so the chakra is called Manipura.

Concentration on this chakra brings control over life and death, the creation of heat, and knowledge of the internal functions of the physical body.

Patanjali Muni describes the experiences that come from the entry of the Kundalini into this chakra:

> "In the navel chakra is knowledge of the workings of the parts of the body."
>
> [*Yoga Sutra*, III-30]

> "From the conquest of the samana comes blazing light and heat."
>
> (Ibid. III-41]

Svadhishthana Chakra

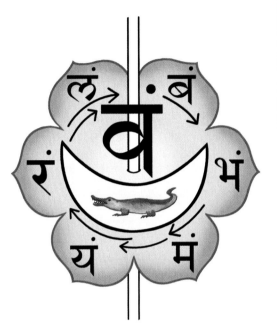

Location	Between navel and genitals
Number of Petals	Six
Color	White
Shape	Crescent
Related Element	Water
Prana-Vayu	Apana
Presiding Deity	Brahma
Quality	Rajas
Seed Letter	Vam वं
Vehicle of Kundalini	Crocodile
Results of Meditation	Control of the element water Control of material desires
***So'Ham Hansaha* Repetitions**	Six thousand

THE NEXT ONE BELOW IS THE SVADHISHTHANA CHAKRA, located between the navel and the genitals. It has six white petals and is crescent shaped. The deity is Brahma. It is related to the water element (liquid). The prana-vayu is apana and the quality rajas. The seed letter is Vam and the vehicle a crocodile. This chakra is the origin of the urge for procreation and is called Svadhishthana (good standing place, well positioned; usually said of a war chariot).

Concentration on this chakra brings control over the water element or the powers of transformation and can bring control over material desires. However, piercing this chakra does cause a great increase in physical desires so it is dangerous and should be crossed over quickly.

Muladhara Chakra

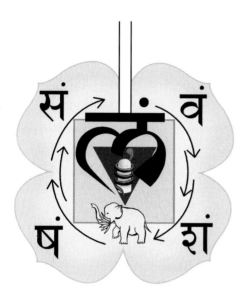

Location	Between anus and genitals
Number of Petals	Four
Color	Yellow
Shape	Square
Related Element	Earth
Prana-Vayu	Apana
Presiding Deity	Ganesha
Quality	Tamas
Seed Letter	Lam लं
Vehicle of Kundalini	Airavata elephant
Results of Meditation	Gain knowledge of scriptures Increase intellect
So'Ham Hansaha Repetitions	Six hundred

FINALLY, BELOW THIS IS THE BASE, the Muladhara chakra, which is also referred to as the *bhuta shringata* (the junction or knot of being) and the *mula shringata* (root junction) in the *Bhuta Shuddhi* mantra.

The Muladhara is located between the anus and the genitals. It has four yellow petals and a square shape. Its element is earth. The prana-vayu is apana, the presiding deity is Ganesha and the quality is *tamas*. The seed letter is Lam and the vehicle is the Airavata, seven-tusked white elephant. Concentration on this chakra brings knowledge of the scriptures and increases the intellect and the ability to write. It also brings knowledge of the earth and the nature of the physical world.

After creation of the Muladhara chakra, the Kundalini goes dormant and rests there. The petals of the chakra hang downwards and are closed. The person's perception of the world is also closed and limited so that one's life feels enclosed in frustration and unhappiness. The awakening of the Kundalini and her reentrance into the spinal column causes the petals to turn upwards as each chakra is penetrated and opened. Because it is the place where the Kundalini lies dormant, this chakra is called Muladhara (root support).

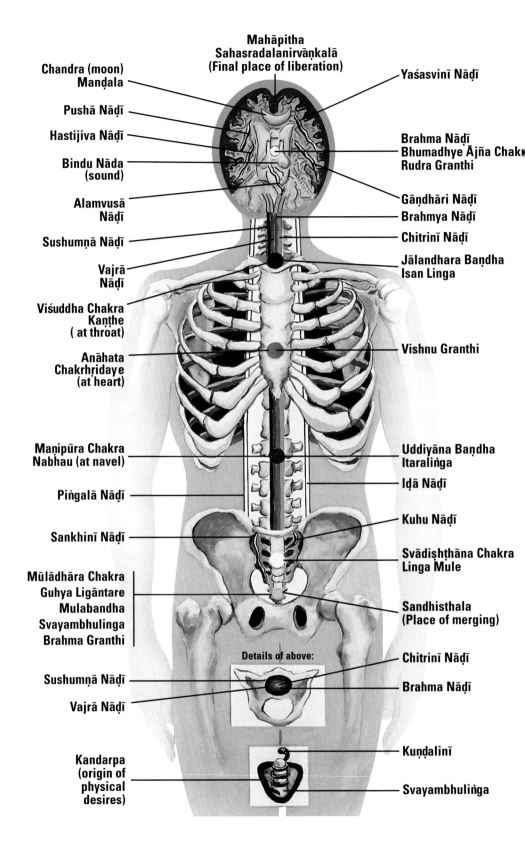

Upon reentering the Sushumna nadi in the spinal cord, the speed of the Kundalini Shakti and the manner of its motion change from chakra to chakra. At times She is deliberate and ponderous like an elephant, at times leaping like a deer or gliding sinuously like a crocodile in water. This motion is described in terms of the various animals called the vehicles of Kundalini.

When the chakras are created, the movement of the Kundalini creates shapes in the form of the letters of the Sanskrit alphabet. These are the bija (seed) mantras at the center of each chakra and on the petals of each lotus. It is by the vibration of this movement that the petals are formed.

There are three *granthi* (knots) in the passageway of the Sushumna nadi, related to the three gunas or qualities. As each knot is untied, the binding quality of its associated guna disappears, leaving finally a state of *turiya* (impersonal spirit) or *nirguna* (of no quality). In the Muladhara is found the Brahma granthi related to rajas-guna. In the Anahata chakra, is the Vishnu granthi related to the sattva-guna and in the Ajna chakra is the Rudra granthi related to tamas-guna.* These granthi may be considered like obstructions blocking the entrance to that chakra to the awakened Kundalini. There are also various deities in each chakra whose precise functions will be discussed at another time.

Similarly, when She is asleep in the Muladhara chakra, the Kundalini Shakti is in the form of a serpent coiled about a *lingam* in three and a half turns, each of the turns representing one of the gunas and the half-turn representing nirguna or turiya.

The *Yoga Sutra* also mentions other benefits that flow from the workings of the Kundalini on the body:

> "From the loosening of the cause of bondage and from knowledge of the wandering currents of the mind (is the power) to enter another body."
>
> [*Yoga Sutra*, III-39]

---

* There is considerable difference of opinion with regard to the granthis. Some sources say that the Brahma granthi is located in the Svadhishthana chakra and the Vishnu granthi in the Vishuddha chakra. In the outline that I have given above, I have followed the *Yoga-Kundalini Upanishad*. This is an area where more research needs to be done to settle these questions through personal experience.

This refers to knowledge of the nadis and chakras.

"From the Kurma nadis, firmness."

[Ibid. III-32]

Here, the specific nadis are mentioned by name (the words "Kurma nadis" appear in the original Sanskrit). They are subsidiary channels in the neck just behind the throat. "Firmness" means the ability to maintain one asana for a long time without moving and also indicates firm control in general.

"From meditation on the relationship between body and space (akasha), one becomes light like a tuft of grass and thus goes into space."

[Ibid. III-43]

In the *Bhagavad Gita*, Lord Krishna says that Maya, the world-creating Shakti of Vishnu, has these three gunas or qualities: sattva, rajas and tamas. These manifest as balance or intelligence, force or passion, and inertia or dullness, respectively. This Maya is very impressive, very energetic and powerful. It binds the world together.

"Divine indeed this guna-creation,
My Maya-illusion difficult to cross over;
Those who truly surrender to Me,
They cross over this Maya."

[*Bhagavad Gita*, Chapter 7, Verse 14]

God says that on one side is his Maya, which keeps all the individual lives bound to this world, to this materialistic life, and on the other side is his *bhakti*, the devotion that grants liberation. They both belong to him. At different times, the forms and methods of devotion change but meditation is the easiest tool. One can reach God very quickly with that. After Shaktipat initiation, once the Kundalini is awakened, She can grant liberation.

Until recently, physical scientists and even psychologists have learned very little about the Kundalini. Like one carefully examining the trunk of an elephant without knowing of the rest of the body, they have not been able to tap the great energy of the chakras of the subtle body.

A great river springs up in the Himalayas, where the rain falls from the heavens, and eventually merges itself in the sea. In its path the flow of the river creates currents that are many times stronger than the flow of the river itself. A ship can sink and the best of swimmers can drown in these currents.

In a similar way, the life force of the Kundalini arises in the Sahasrara at the top of the head and ends in the Muladhara chakra below the base of the spine. In her path the Kundalini creates the six chakras like currents or whirlpools in a river. Just as the currents of a river are stronger than the flow of the river itself, so the energy levels in the chakras are of a much higher intensity than the energy of the steady flow of the Kundalini.

At the Ajna chakra the energy flow divides into three nadis or channels. Along the two sides of the spine are the nadis *Ida* (on the left) and *Pingala* (on the right), with the *Sushumna* nadi down the center. In the ordinary living being, the life forces flow through the Ida and Pingala, and the Sushumna is closed. Their effects are variously concentrated in the five lower chakras so that worldly activities may go on. The sixth, or Ajna, chakra is the dwelling place of the *Atma* (soul) in its purest state as a separated and individualized life form.

Within the yellow cube of the Muladhara chakra between the rectum and the genitals, there is a triangular shaped place where the dormant Kundalini is coiled around the *Svayambhu-lingam*. The lingam is a form of Shiva, and Svayambhu literally means "own-going-being" or what God is in his own being. The place is called Sumeru after the mountain that represents the axis of a universe. The Kundalini there is like a subtle form of static electricity. This area is very delicate and can produce intense emotional feelings. Yogis have discovered that whenever a person has intense emotional feelings (which may be devotional, or may involve just high thinking, or be related to accidental gains of pain or pleasure), then this area is affected and becomes hot immediately.

This is proof that the Kundalini is coiled here, and whenever there is a flow of intense emotional feelings it strikes against this area, affecting it and causing it to produce heat.

In order to carry on the activities of the world, desires are formed here and it is through this area that male and female unite in sexual intercourse to procreate despite all their conflicts in life. During sadhana it is helpful to retain the energies spent on sexual relations so that they may be used for spiritual development. In order not to waste these energies *brahmacharis* (celibates) wear a loincloth.

After forming the Muladhara chakra and assuming the form of a serpent, the Kundalini goes to sleep facing downwards, closing the door to the Sushumna nadi. The nature of all subtle energies is to move in a circular path. Kundalini too, after returning to her origin, coils up in a circular fashion. She continues to be active as long as the activities of nature operate.

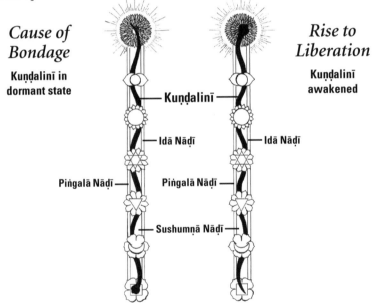

Cause of Bondage

Kuṇḍalinī in dormant state

— Kuṇḍalinī —

Rise to Liberation

Kuṇḍalinī awakened

— Idā Nāḍī
Idā Nāḍī —

Piṅgalā Nāḍī —   Piṅgalā Nāḍī —

— Sushumṇā Nāḍī —

Through experimentation yogis have learned how to turn this energy away from going around and around in these coiling circles so that it turns upward and enters the Sushumna nadi. Then, instead of creating bondage, it grants liberation. When the Kundalini Shakti starts Her travel from the base of the spinal column, the individual rises higher and higher in spiritual insight. One's life is fulfilled. When She reaches the brain center from which She started, then the individual reaches liberation, understands one's true identity and attains eternal happiness. The student's spiritual evolution depends directly on this upward travel of the Kundalini. After She reaches the crown chakra, the mind of the practitioner is always peaceful.

Thus, the Kundalini works in two ways. As long as worldly concerns are dominant She causes further bondage, but once She is awakened and enters the Sushumna She grants liberation. All of the samskaras — the ideas, attitudes and habits that mark an individual person — are embedded in the pattern of flow of this Kundalini energy. Even when we see unimaginable visions in dreams, these are just the samskaras, the mind impressions from our past births, operating. They are part of the flow of the Kundalini Herself.

A river flowing from the mountains to the sea can cause great destruction to farms and cities if it floods without control. But if the same floodwaters can be scientifically controlled by dams and distributed by canals, they can irrigate thousands of acres of land, generate electricity and be useful in many ways. Its formerly destructive power can be put to good and constructive use.

Similarly, if the life force of the Kundalini Shakti is controlled and made to flow through the huge, river-like Sushumna nadi, then various types of joy can be experienced and many doors to peace and happiness are opened. The joy felt when the Kundalini reaches the Sahasrara is many times more intense than any kind of physical sensation. This is called the yoga, or union, of jiva and Shiva. There is no greater joy than this merging of the individual life with God.

It is a strict universal law that on any spiritual path, whether undertaken consciously or unconsciously, unless the Kundalini is somehow awakened, no benefits of any kind can be obtained. Whether by devotion or knowledge, by renunciation or divine grace, by austerities or by Shaktipat, when the Kundalini is awakened and begins Her journey home through the Sushumna, then all spiritual experiences can be attained. Many disciples have visions of deities; many get answers from within. Some persons who do japa, or mantra repetition, for a long time finally get visions and do not know that their Kundalini has been awakened, although it has been. Only when the Kundalini is awakened can such experiences occur. This is a fixed law.

As I mentioned before, the Earth is balanced around its axis through the North and South poles by the attraction and repulsion of the positive and negative forces that are continually operating. So too in the human body the forces operating between the Sahasrara and the Muladhara are responsible for maintaining and controlling the body and function as the main control center. These two chakras are the poles of various human experiences such as knowledge, joy, misery, etc. For this reason the Muladhara and the Sahasrara are very important chakras. Many emotional kriyas also begin in the Sahasrara.

In the ordinary human being these currents flow through the Ida and the Pingala, and the mind is distracted and externally oriented. Yogis direct their feeling and emotional currents through the Sushumna to the head, and their minds turn inward instead of being externally directed.

As long as the mind is oriented outside you cannot gain any success in spiritual work. Gohrakhnath, a great saint in India, said, "As long as you can not focus and concentrate your mind, any type of work in this world is useless. You may wear saffron-colored clothes or dress all in white, you may do a lot of austerities and penance, but unless your mind is concentrated, it is all of no use." You must first win over your mind—all else is secondary. As long as you cannot win over your mind, you may try to control your senses by not talking or seeing or hearing, but all that is useless if you cannot keep your mind calm. Until your mind becomes one-pointed, all such efforts are of no avail. If you try to fast but are always thinking about food, it is of no great benefit.

> "The sense objects turn away from the abstinent man leaving the taste; the taste also turns away, when he has seen the Supreme."
>
> [*Bhagavad Gita*, Chap. 2, Verse 59]

Many people say that one should go away to the forest or to the mountains and live the life of a recluse for spiritual growth, but unless it is detached, your mind is going with you and will keep thinking about things back home. It is no good to go to the forest and keep thinking about your friends and family. It is better to live with them and train your mind to be detached from them. That is the real yogi. If, while you are living in society, you direct your thinking toward God and believe that you are "So Ham," that is, a part of Him, an atom of Him, your mind will become detached and concentrated.

When the Kundalini awakens, She passes through the Sushumna and pierces the chakras one by one. If She reaches the Sahasrara, then the big problem is resolved by itself. The mind, turned inward by the great energy and drawn up the Sushumna, becomes automatically one-pointed and concentrated. There is so much energy liberated that nothing in this world remains impossible to do. That is to say, when one has control over the prana-vayu, the currents of vital energy, one is the master of the entire world. The rays of the Sun diffuse gently all over the surface of the world, but if concentrated with a lens they can start a fire. Yogis believe that if the sunrays falling on only 60 acres of land could be collected they would provide energy sufficient to run all the factories in the world. Nowadays, science is working on ways to tap those energies, and I hope they will be successful.

Likewise, if we can tap the powers of our intellect and concentrate them internally, then so much energy is created that no task remains impossible. On the contrary, any work can then be done with great ease. Finally, by the awakening of the Kundalini and the realization of the union of God and the individual living being, the darkness of ignorance is eliminated and one is free.

In the Upanishads it is written that, "Upon reaching the higher levels, the knot of ignorance is loosened, all doubts are eliminated and all karmic bondage is destroyed."

In the sixth chapter of the *Shri Jnaneshwari Gita*, eight kinds of *pranayama* (breathing exercises aimed at controlling energies through controlling the breath) are mentioned, and three kinds of *bandha* for closing temporarily various channels of the energy flow. These are the *mula bandha*, for stopping energy from going past the Muladhara chakra, *udayana bandha* for stopping energy flow at the navel, and *jalandhara bandha* for cutting off the energy flow at the level of the throat. According to Shri Jnaneshwar Maharaj, when pranayama is done together with these bandhas, it will be perfected.

"When yogis practice mula bandha for long periods of time heat is created in the body and the apana vayu, instead of going downward and passing out of the body through the rectum, turns upward and goes towards the stomach. It produces some activity in the stomach and intestines, creating a type of sound. By spreading around in the stomach, it removes excess mucous there, cleansing it. By purifying the seven materials of the body, it destroys excess fat and often eliminates diseases by removing their causes. At that time, due to the heat of the mixing of prana and apana, the Kundalini that was dormant and coiled becomes awakened and straight and eats up the impurities in the disciple's body. After removing wastes of various sorts, it settles in the heart chakra and removes all of the air below it. Then, from the feet up to the head, it finishes removing all of the impurities from every part of the body. Then the yogi's body becomes very dry. The elements of earth and water become purified and dried. Then the energy enters the spinal column, emitting nectar from its mouth and the body of the yogi receives nutrition. Finally, the Kundalini comes to the Ajna chakra and drops nectar there so that the yogi's body is brightened and rejuvenated, getting a sort of luster. Such a yogi receives several powers and after self-realization becomes victorious."

The Kundalini can also be awakened by attaining perfection in the asanas or physical postures of hatha yoga, by pranayama, by God's grace, by meditation or by intense devotion.

Another technique of awakening the Kundalini is Shaktipat, the transmission of power. A powerful yogi can transmit energy to the disciple in any one of four ways: by touch, gaze, words or thought. He may touch the disciple and transmit the energy through physical contact, or gaze at the disciple and let the energy flow through his eyes. The yogi may utter words or mantric sounds as the carriers of the energy or, more subtly, he may do it directly by mere thought. Of course, he may also use any combination of these methods.

Only those yogis who have complete control over the prana, the energy of the subtle body, can perform Shaktipat. This help is of immense value.

Their guidance and example help to keep the disciple on the correct path, and from time to time their energy can give fresh impulse to the disciple's Kundalini and help eliminate obstructions and blockages that may occur.

Once the Kundalini is awakened the disciple begins to get various experiences, like flashes of light, visions, bodily movements and vibrations called kriyas, intense feelings of devotion, increased emotionalism, etc. Different individuals have different experiences, and there is no particular pattern applicable to everyone. Then, if the disciple persists in spiritual practice and meditation, the Kundalini travels upward through the Sushumna, piercing each chakra in succession, and finally reaches the Sahasrara.

As long as the Kundalini is dormant, the individual spends an unhappy, unfulfilled life, bound by his limited perception. When the Kundalini is awakened and traveling upward, the disciple develops deeper and deeper spiritual insight and his life is more and more fulfilled. When the Kundalini completes her return to the Sahasrara, the disciple perceives one's true identity, attains liberation, and is established in eternal happiness. Spiritual knowledge—as distinguished from mere book knowledge—depends directly on this upward movement of the Kundalini.

Now, a few words about meditation and the breath. Of all the forms of meditation, meditation through attention on the breath is probably the easiest and most direct method. By doing pranayama in conjunction with meditation the disciple can coordinate and integrate the various energy systems, and learn how to get control over the prana. That, in turn, leads to control over the mind, which brings unique joy and peace. The person realizes that the entire world is the creation of one God. If that happens on a large scale, the miseries of the world will end and there will be peace and happiness everywhere.

Self-realization is the ultimate and most desirable state to be attained. Although the awakened Kundalini leads to that state, there is no guarantee that it will be attained in one lifetime, though the awakening does very substantially hasten the process of that evolution. It is encouraging to know that there are many, quite tangible, side benefits gained even during the early stages of the awakening of the Kundalini and Her upward travel. The health of the disciple improves. His skin and body become more attractive, and his voice becomes rich and sweet. Body odor is reduced and wastes substantially decrease. He feels light and energetic and his mind becomes rested and peaceful. Many diseases of body and mind are automatically eliminated. This is all due to the general purification effect of the Kundalini on both body and mind. Diseases caused by irregularities in the flow of prana are gradually eliminated. At more advanced levels, these benefits are intensified and encompass subtler realms. The disciple achieves peace and mental control, becomes creative, develops a profound understanding of nature, and enjoys inner bliss. He becomes a strong individual, a complete person, and is able to function in adverse circumstances with great poise. He learns to consciously draw prana from the universe and how to use it to cure mental and physical diseases in him and others. Ultimately, of course, he encounters total reality, the absolute truth and knowledge of the Self.

At this stage, I would like to point out that spiritual evolution can not take place unless the Kundalini is awakened. There are many spiritual disciplines and techniques that do not aim at directly awakening the Kundalini. However, the Kundalini must be aroused if there is to be any spiritual progress. Thus, if any discipline is successful that means it has awakened the Kundalini, at least in an indirect way. The practitioner of the discipline may not even recognize the fact that his progress and experiences are the result of the functioning of the Kundalini. Nevertheless, the Kundalini does keep working and is the source of his enlightenment. Once the Kundalini is awakened, She does not become dormant again. She will try to execute her upward progress all the time and will keep the aspirant on the spiritual path, giving one the protection and encouragement that one needs.

Finally, I must add a warning against attempting to directly arouse the Kundalini without the aid and protection of a competent guru. One would not attempt to build a high building without an engineer and an architect, and this path of spiritual development is just as complex, just as filled with opportunities to make disastrous errors. After Shaktipat, as my disciples know, I am always with them and they need have no fear of misstep, but one entering this area without a teacher is like an untrained city person who wanders off into the jungle alone.

God always sends a guru to those who are ready and need one. When the time is ripe, the teacher appears. You may search for a guru or not search, as you wish, but one will come along when he is needed. Your feelings will tell you who is the correct teacher. Trust them and when your guru appears, accept his teachings.

Different teachers have different styles of talking and use various differing methods. This is because different people have different needs. Ultimately, all true teachers are one. I spread a banquet for my disciples where they may eat until they are satisfied. If you are hungry, come, meditate and experience for yourself.

The awakening of the Kundalini, the realization of the Self and the subsequent practice of the controlled use of these energies for the benefit of others is Shakti Yoga, or Kundalini Maha Yoga.

Sarve Bhavantu Sukhinah	Let everyone, everywhere, be happy.
Sarve Santu Niramayah	Let everyone be healthy.
Sarve Bhadrani Pashyantu	Let everyone see good fortune
Ma Kaschid Dukhabhag Bhavet.	and never be filled with suffering.

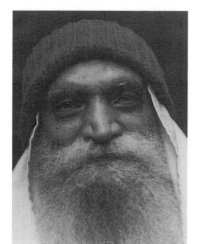

Questions and Answers

This chapter is taken from various Satsang sessions with Shri Dhyanyogiji and disciples. Satsang, which means "in the company of Truth", is a question and answer session in which students pose questions to the Master. This is a traditional teaching method in this and other yogic paths.

Disciple (D): Why does a person meditate? Why do they need it?

Guruji (G): Why do you eat? Just as food is nourishment for the body, so meditation is nourishment for the soul. It is a way to find out who you really are. There are many advantages. Your mind becomes exhilarated. You gain greater peace of mind and relaxation. Your concentration increases. You gain a sense of oneness that you feel will increase, not intellectually but spiritually. Meditation is not only food for the soul but for the universe. It also increases efficiency of your day-to-day activities. Everything is better if you meditate.

D: What is the function of meditation? Can one enter the higher states of consciousness without meditation?

G: There is no escape from it. It may vary from one individual to another with respect to time. Some may pass through it very quickly, some more slowly. It depends on the previous mind impressions and previous karma. There is only one physiological way in which *dhyana,* or meditation, will start, and that is through the opening of the Sushumna nadi. There are many ways this can occur, but if it does not occur then nothing will happen. It could happen through extreme joy, extreme distress, through devotion, or through the grace of God or Guru. This must take place, whatever the race or nationality of the meditator. Everyone has to pass through this process.

D: What is *dhyana* (meditation)?

G: I will use the example of this watch. As long as you are aware of the process of concentration on the watch, you know you are there. You know the watch is there, and you know that you are concentrating on the watch. When it becomes dhyana, you lose track of the fact that you are concentrating on the watch. You remain there, the watch remains there, but you do not know that you are concentrating on the watch. The next step is that you lose track of yourself also. You don't know that you are concentrating on the watch. There is just the watch. That is samadhi.

D: What is *tamas samadhi?*

G: There are three types of samadhi. All are good but some are better. If you are hungry you can have dried bread, which is satisfying to some extent, or you can have a full meal that is much better than just dried bread. In tamas samadhi you go into a state like sleep and don't feel your experiences. Later you will have light and other experiences.

D: What are *pratyahara, dharna, dhyana* and *samadhi?*

G: As they apply to the practice of meditation, they have special meanings. Pratyahara means withdrawal of the senses and mind. Dharna means to direct your consciousness towards one thing while maintaining awareness of the outside world. Dhyana is awareness of the object and the self only. Samadhi is where the self is forgotten and it is merged in oneness with the object of concentration.

D: What is *sadhana*?

G: It is spiritual practice and meditation on the spiritual path.

D: What is *Maha Yoga*?

G: Literally, "Maha" means great, and yoga you know. Kundalini Yoga, Maha Yoga and Raja Yoga are all names for Kundalini Maha Yoga. In each path the Kundalini awakens in your body and reaches the Sahasrara chakra. They are called by different names, but they are the same. They are practices of meditation along different lines, but the ultimate goal is the same.

D: Is this Kundalini Maha Yoga different from meditation?

G: No. They are one and the same. Meditation is an instrument. There are various ways of practicing yoga, and meditation is one of these techniques.

D: What is the highest point one can go during meditation?

G: To the Sahasrara chakra.

D: Is everything there as you look?

G: Yes. Whatever is in your body becomes the universe, and the result is indescribable joy.

D: Is there more than one universe?

G: There are so many universes, they cannot be counted.

D: If you reach the Sahasrara chakra, are you the lord of a universe?

G: It is the Ultimate. It is nothing like being the lord or a king. It is more; it is peace of mind, complete knowledge, a state of perfect balance, a feeling of oneness with God. There is nothing; no sky, no Moon, no Sun.

Once you are there you never want to return. When you reach the highest goal, there is nothing more to achieve.

D: Does this type of meditation lead to God in the way of Buddha or Christ?

G: We are made of the same basic elements as they are. As they reached oneness with God, so can we. This is one of the paths that can lead to this oneness. Every human being can become one with God by proper sadhana, which includes meditation as one of the main aspects. If a plane can take the President from New York to Paris, it can take you there also. Spiritual sadhana has the same possibilities for everyone.

D: What is happening when someone goes into a deep meditation?

G: What happens when you go to sleep? It is difficult to narrate to a person who has not slept. When you are in a deep meditation you experience purposeless joy. You feel as if you've taken a dive in the ocean of joy. You must experience it to know what it is like.

D: Is it dangerous? Is there a chance a person will not come out of it?

G: No.

D: Do we need to go into a deep meditation to consider it a good meditation?

G: When you're eating and you feel satisfied with your food, do you need to do anything to know the satisfaction? As we get butter from milk, and ghee from the butter, all you need to do is start with milk.

D: Do you mean to just keep "plugging along"?

G: That's right.

D: Sometimes I have what appears to be a poor meditation, but after it's over I feel spaced and stoned. Why is that?

G: When you start eating, you do not know when you will feel satisfied. When you have finished eating and are satisfied, you know it. When a yogi experiences transcendental consciousness, he feels oneness with everything and goes into a state of samadhi. Once he reaches this state, no matter what calamities befall him, he is happy with that consciousness. You are all on the same path going towards that same goal. You don't have to worry.

D: Why is it easy to get into a deep meditation at some times and not others? Does it have anything to do with the length of time since eating?

G: If you have a full stomach, it is not good for meditation. If a hose is full of water, nothing more can be put into it. With an empty stomach the energy channels are empty, and so the energy can flow through.

D: Is it all right to drink water before meditation?

G: If you feel thirsty, drink water. Then you should wait half an hour before meditation. If you are hungry, eat a little food, but don't meditate for at least an hour. Ordinarily, after eating a meal, one should wait two and one half-hours before meditating.

D: Since initiation I find that I haven't been able to meditate at all.

G: Were you able to meditate before?

D: Yes. Now I don't know if I am meditating or not.

G: It comes by practice. Keep trying. When meditating just keep your attention on your breath. Don't think whether you are getting into it or not.

One disciple in India came to meditation every day and complained that he couldn't get into meditation. He would not close his eyes, but would keep on watching the *kriyas* of others. I asked him if he closed his eyes while meditating. He replied, "No, I keep on observing people."

If you were sitting with others at a meal and you observed what they eat rather than eating yourself, would you be satisfied? If the nuts and bolts of an engine were not fitted properly, would the engine start? If you have a bank account and don't write checks on it, will it be any use to you? Similarly, when trying to meditate, if you don't close your eyes you won't be able to enjoy the meditation. The joy of meditation is inside, not outside. It is not like going to a movie. When you go to a movie, you must keep your eyes open and watch, but here you have to close your eyes and watch inside. Only then will you get into meditation. As a machine will work only if the nuts and bolts are properly fitted, so closing the eyes will get you into meditation.

The next day the disciple started closing his eyes and was able to meditate. You are all instructed to close your eyes and mentally watch your breath. Then you will get into meditation. If you want to fill a pot with milk that already contains water, you have to empty it first. Similarly, by cutting yourself off from external activities, you can fill yourself with inner joy.

D: When distracting thoughts come in the middle of meditation, what can we do about them?

G: Become an observer of all your thoughts. Do not think you are the thoughts and do not make any value judgments about them. Just be a third person observer. When you sit down for a meal, other thoughts continue. You may think about going shopping, but you don't immediately jump up and go to the store. So while meditating other thoughts may come, but just go on with the meditation. Eventually the thoughts will stop.

D: What should I do when my mind is wandering?

G: When a child does not want to take medicine, you hold his nose to make him open his mouth. When you want to make a boat stop drifting about, you drop an anchor. So it is with your mind. It needs to be anchored.

There is nothing wrong with the mind moving around in itself, but the mind is like a two-edged sword. The mind is the cause of both bondage and liberation. It depends on which way you want to go. The way to control it is a great art and a great science. You must learn it slowly. Technically, your prana begins to move in the Sushumna instead of the side nadis, the Ida and Pingala. Then the mind is concentrated and you get more control. The technique is to put the mind into that mold, and that is something to be learned. For example, you can learn to cook a special dish but if you don't experiment, you will not be able to do it. The same is true here. You cannot learn it in books. You must experiment, practice and learn it from the right people. Then you can make progress.

D: Does the process of the Kundalini continue even if the mind wanders and you do not surrender?

G: When you try to meditate and the *Mantrochar* recording is playing (The Mantrochar is the collection of mantras that Shri Dhyanyogiji chants during meditation.), the energy is working. Sometimes it may be deep; sometimes you may come out of it. Going in and out means that the energy is working and leading to greater concentration. Anything new takes time. Practice is necessary. This principle is true on the spiritual path, too. Eventually you will have more concentration.

D: I would like to know how to improve my meditation. I feel peaceful and quiet, but sometimes I feel that I am falling asleep. I do not know if I am meditating.

G: You are lucky. Lots of millionaires cannot sleep. They are prepared to spend thousands of dollars, but nothing can put them to sleep. When you are trying to get to the ocean, initially you may find stones and mud, but once you get into deeper waters you will be able to float. The feeling of peace is a sign of getting into meditation and is called *tamas dhyana*. It is a good sign.

D: When we meditate should we meditate on something special?

G: The best thing to meditate on is your own breathing. That is the closest thing to you and it helps make your mind one-pointed.

D: This morning during meditation we concentrated on breathing, and I couldn't go beyond counting eight. Then I lapsed into space. I was no longer aware of counting. Then I would remember, try again and maybe get to three. The same thing happened several times.

G: That is a deep meditation, so there was no need for counting. If you want to use incense, you take a match and light it, and then you don't need the match any more. It was only for lighting the incense. In the same way, counting is for concentrating the mind, making it peaceful, and achieving oneness. If you have concentration, there is no need to count. This is a good sign.

D: How long during the day should I meditate?

G: As long as you enjoy it without getting physically tired or mentally bored. One to one-and-one-half hours a day is a good amount of time.

D: As I get more involved in sadhana, it becomes increasingly difficult to go out and work in the world. Do you have any suggestions?

G: If there were a rain of dollars in your home, it would be up to you to decide if you wanted to keep them or throw them away. Slowly you will be able to attain a balance between the two, and such a balance is recommended.

D: Is there such a thing as practicing too much meditation? Will things change too fast?

G: Suppose a doctor gives you a medicine to take for ten days and you finish it in two days. What happens? What would happen if there was enough food for ten days and you finished it in two? Everything should be done within limits, and that is why one needs a guru.

D: When I first started meditating it was unproductive, but now I want to do nothing but meditate.

G: You must maintain balance, and you need guidance. If it is done in a balanced way you will progress, but you must be in balance.

D: In a group meditation, if someone goes into a deep meditation, are there any instructions about how to bring the person out of it? Or should one let it take care of itself?

G: The person will wake up automatically. If you want to bring them out of the deep meditation, wait until there is a little movement. It can be dangerous if there is no movement at all. No one will die because of a deep meditation. In a deep meditation, the body becomes youthful and disease disappears. Many yogis in the Himalayas are alone, and they go into a deep meditation with no one to bring them out of it. In deep meditation there is not hunger or thirst, just joy. The heart and breathing are very slow.

D: Is there a danger if someone awakens you because of not understanding about deep meditations?

G: A person should be awakened slowly. If it is too sudden, it can affect the heart. In a deep meditation the heart is very slow, so a quick push can affect it. Ordinarily, the heart beats 72 times a minute, but in a deep meditation it is only four or five. A doctor would say that the person is on the verge of a collapse. Really it is just a state of joy.

D: Is an "out of body" state the same as a deep meditation?

G: That comes after crossing over the stage of deep meditation.

D: Could a sudden noise, such as a dog barking or a telephone ringing, have the same bad effect as a physical push?

G: Yes. That is why yogis in India use caves for meditation. You should have a peaceful place to meditate, especially if you go into a deep meditation.

D: When I am in a deep meditation state, but aware, where am I? What's happening?

G: You are everywhere and nowhere. That you are aware you are in deep meditation means that you are in the deep meditation. It means that you are in your own heart. The place for the soul is the heart chakra. From this place you have this experience. The soul has several different offices, but its place of residence is the heart.

D: Why do we concentrate on the third eye chakra?

G: That is the way to the soul. The third eye is an office, but the heart is the place of residence. The third eye is the way to the goal. Any of the six chakras can be used for concentration. Even outside objects like the sun or the moon or a beautiful sight can be used for concentration. The important thing is concentration on something. If your mind is concentrated on anything, the rest comes easier. If your mind is not concentrated, then all other techniques are useless. You can put on saffron robes, renounce the world and be withdrawn from worldly affairs, but all these will not work until your mind becomes concentrated. You may practice austerities like fasting, but if your mind is always thinking of food, what use is it? You can go to churches or temples or holy places, but if your mind is wandering to the city or job or the home, what good is it? You may be celibate, but if your mind is wandering to sexual activities, then what use is it? Until you control the mind the external means are of no use. If you go to the Himalayas, sit in a cave and try to meditate, but your mind is back home thinking about your family or business, then that is useless. Wherever you go, your mind goes with you. Until the boat is anchored, until the mind is controlled, there will be problems. It is not necessary to leave your home and family to achieve concentration. You should stay where you are and do it there. The external means are difficult. It is better to use the chakras in your body for concentration. It will be a lot easier to concentrate there than on external things.

D: Can I meditate on the heart chakra during meditation?

G: Yes, you can. The third eye is easier for concentration, though, because we are used to seeing through the two eyes. There is no need to concentrate on different centers. For instance, you cannot eat all the fruit in this bowl at once. You eat one at a time. You cannot concentrate on all chakras all of the time. If you have control of one center, then controlling all centers becomes very easy.

D: When you concentrate on the third eye, is there something else you should visualize, like a light?

G: No. You don't have to visualize anything there. By concentrating the light will come automatically.

D: The chakras are inside, so how do we concentrate on things we cannot see?

G: We see with our two eyes, but if you close your eyes and think you are seeing in the middle of your two eyes, then it will be easy. By doing this you will be able to start concentrating more and more. When the Sushumna door opens and prana enters there, the real progress will begin. Everyone is used to seeing with his or her eyes. It is easier to transfer the attention to the center between the eyes with the eyes closed. Then you can look inwards and the act of concentration becomes possible. The third eye chakra is the easiest one to concentrate on. Once you are able to concentrate on this chakra, then it is possible to concentrate on the other chakras as well.

D: Are there any negative side effects from concentrating too much on one chakra?

G: Concentrating on any of the chakras does not involve any negative energy whatsoever. If you overdo it you might have some physical problems because of too much energy concentration. Depending on your capacity, which varies from person to person, if you can concentrate on one chakra for a longer time, that is good. Otherwise, you just keep on concentrating on any of the chakras for the time you can do so without any physical contradictions. It is like a plate with different kinds of food. You do not eat everything together; you eat them one at a time. Similarly, concentrating on the chakras one after another is more helpful.

D: What of people who have negative experiences with the Kundalini?

G: When you practice Kundalini Yoga, it should be with guidance. Otherwise it could be difficult. If you have no guidance and do not know how to prepare certain medicines, you may kill the patient. There are a lot of medicines. If you were sick you could experiment with them and take a chance, or you could go to a doctor who knows which to prescribe. It is better to take them from a person who knows.

D: Why do you ask us to do deep breathing before meditation?

G: Deep breathing brings the mind back from external activity. When a kite flies in an unsteady wind, you pull the string to steady it. It is the same with the deep breathing; it steadies the mind and makes it easier to concentrate in meditation.

D: Is it all right to chant "Om" while meditating?

G: Yes, but it is better to concentrate on the breath rather than the vibration. The breath itself will have a rhythm that gets one deeper into meditation. The chanting will stop when you go deeper. If you work to keep chanting even when you are deep, it will shake the mind. Then it is better to stop. When the chanting stops automatically it is a very good sign.

D: If one goes into meditation without following the breath or concentrating on the third eye, is that all right?

G: These are all techniques so that you can begin to meditate, but if you are already in meditation then you do not require them. It is all right just to meditate in that case. It is like when you are boarding an aircraft and there is a ladder you have to climb up. Some people will step on each step to reach the aircraft. Some might skip two or three steps. The main thing is that you board the aircraft and fly. It is not important how many steps you go through. These are just instruments you make use of to reach your goal.

D: How many levels of meditation are there?

G: Six levels, corresponding to the six chakras.

D: Which is preferable, to meditate on the breath and count "Om" or "Ram", or to use the Guru mantra given at the time of initiation?

G: Whether you say "Ram" or the Guru mantra, once your breath becomes rhythmic, then you become one-pointed. When you get angry, do hard labor or run, your breathing becomes rapid. When you are emotional, your breathing is irregular. When the mind is wavering over something, the breath is also irregular. Until the breath is regular you cannot get into deep meditation because the mind and prana are related. If the breath is regular, the mind will also be regular. If you breathe naturally, without emotional or mental disturbance, the mind will become regular. If your mantra is such that it can become part of the breath, it helps to regularize the breath. If it is long or complicated, the breath cannot become regular.

Those who sing know that if there is a disturbance in the rhythm, they do not enjoy the singing. So if the rhythm is lost, the joy is lost. "Ram" is a short mantra and it accords with the breath to help make it regular. The mind comes back to itself and can become concentrated.

61

If a person has two legs he can walk properly. If one of the legs is lost, it is as if he has lost both legs. He cannot walk. Similarly, if either the mind or prana is controlled, it is as if both are controlled. "Ram" is easy for this purpose, or you may say "God" or "Christ" if you like. It is one and the same.

D: Would it be beneficial physically and spiritually to chant "Ram" while jogging or working?

G: Certainly.

D: Before Shaktipat initiation, I was practicing pranayama through the mouth. Now you tell me to do deep breathing through the nose. As I listen during meditation I hear every different type of breathing. What is the proper way, and what is the benefit of breathing through the nose as opposed to the mouth?

G: All animals, including man, naturally breathe through the nose. Breathing through the nose helps prevent bacteria from entering the lungs because of the mucous and hairs. By breathing through the mouth there is more strain on the lungs, and a larger possibility of bacteria entering the lungs. In none of the Yoga scriptures does it say to breathe through the mouth. There is no yogi in India who teaches this. Those people who practice it contract diseases and can develop stomach problems.

It is good for you to breathe through the nose. If you are trying to enter a house through the proper door, it is easy. Trying to enter by breaking through a wall is a tough job. The mouth is for eating, and the nose is for breathing. What would happen if you tried to eat through your nose? There are rules of nature that we must follow. Feet are made for walking, so if you try to walk on your hands it is very difficult. If you try to write with your feet, it may be possible, but very hard to do.

Any vehicle, like a car or a plane, starts slowly and then gradually speeds up. Even if we walk or run, we gradually take on more speed. If an engine jumps when starting, it means there is some defect. Engines pick up speed slowly. Similarly, a person who is beginning to do pranayama should start off slowly. When strength develops, then it is possible to go faster. As you gain practice, and your breathing system becomes strong enough, you will be able to do it quickly. Fast pranayama quickly affects the mind, bringing it within. A beginner cannot start doing fast pranayama. Begin with deep, slow breathing, and then increase the speed.

D: I have been told that breathing through the mouth activates the throat chakra. I don't feel this when I breathe through the nose.

G: At first, when you breathe through the nose, it feels shallow. When you practice, you will be able to breathe fast and deep. This is what works best. The effect of this breathing is like a tortoise going into its shell— the mind goes within and becomes one-pointed. Thoughts stop. Do whatever is convenient to you, but remember that the basic idea is that breath should be from deep down in order to work.

As you mentioned, breathing through the mouth does work on certain chakras, but it is not good in the long run. Suppose you drink milk through the nose. It will reach your stomach, but it is not natural and will eventually cause damage. By breathing through the mouth, the Kundalini may be awakened but it is like entering a house by breaking through a wall. The whole building may eventually be damaged.

D: How many times a day can I do pranayama? I have been doing it three times a day for 30 minutes.

G: Do not practice pranayama until two and one half-hours after a meal. Before a meal you can do it. If you have had something to drink then you should wait for half an hour. If you sit for meditation after pranayama it will be helpful. Morning and evening are the best times.

D: I have met several competent yogis who teach a type of cooling pranayama done through the mouth to aid digestion and sleep. What do you think of it?

G: In this type of pranayama, the tongue should curl upwards at the sides and air should flow over the tongue and come out through the nose. This is cooling on the system if you are hot. It is not the same as breathing through the mouth. This is a technique that takes very little air through the mouth and is not damaging if you practice it within your capacity. This pranayama is for the special purpose of cooling, and is not for using anytime. There are many kinds of pranayama for different purposes. One is floating on water for hours, but it is not recommended for meditation. There are eight basic types of pranayama. *Puraka, rechaka, kumbhaka* and *bhastrika* are recommended.

D: Is bhastrika breath as effective as the method you teach?

G: Yes. Mild bhastrika is suggested. It is not damaging.

D: I was doing pranayama for a while, but I was in the city in heavy polluted air and it did not feel good, so I quit. Can such air be damaging in pranayama?

G: When doing sadhana it is necessary to have clean air. Once you have attained your goal, it doesn't matter. Use the fresh air of the morning and evening.

D: What is the function of the Mantrochar? How does it work and how was it developed?

G: The Rishis in India developed mantras a long time ago. They put these chants together in a particular way in order to produce specific effects. It is not so much the meaning of the chants, but the sound vibration and the precise rhythm in which they are spoken that has the effect.

D: The Mantrochar is in the Sanskrit language, but here people only understand English. Is the language and meaning important to understand?

G: The sound is the important part. It creates the vibrations and it will affect everyone whether they understand the meaning or not. It is better if they understand the meaning, but even if they don't understand, the sound will work because the vibrations will affect all.

D: I sleep during the Mantrochar and then I can't sleep for the rest of the night.

G: Maybe you get all the rest you need in one hour. One hour of deep yogic sleep is equivalent to eight hours of regular sleep. You should do *japa* for the rest of the time.

D: If a person goes to sleep during the Mantrochar is it all right?

G: That is all right, you can sleep. That will relax and rejuvenate the body and mind, but this should not be your final objective. The final objective is Self-realization and God-realization. By listening to the Mantrochar during meditation and doing japa, the realization will come.

D: What can an aspirant do to diminish the need for sleep and to wake up early to do sadhana?

G: Before going to sleep, pray to me to wake you up at a certain time, and I will work as your alarm clock.

D: Is it all right to use a mantra that I have been saying to get into meditation, or should I use the mantra I was given at initiation?

G: If it is more convenient for you to use the mantra you are used to, you can go ahead with that. The mantra that I have given you will come automatically. So don't worry. You can go ahead with whatever is coming to you now.

65

D: What is unique about the "Ram" meditation compared to others?

G: The names of all the Gods are basically the same, but this one is short. "Ra" is said with the mouth open; "m" with the mouth closed. Bad things go out when the mouth is open, and closing the mouth keeps them out. "R" stands for creation; "A" for the sustenance of creation; and "M" stands for the destruction of creation. It represents all of existence.

D: When repeating the Bhuta Shuddhi mantra, how do I know when I've gone into meditation?

G: When the time comes for meditation, you yourself will know. You will forget you are saying a mantra, and you will feel you are going into meditation. Every day you go to bed to go to sleep and you do this automatically. No one tells you when you go to sleep. You know by yourself. So in meditation you also know by yourself.

D: Can you substitute meditation for exercise? If the mind controls the body and I exercise the mind in meditation, can I substitute this for physical exercise?

G: It can be done but it is very difficult. The physical and the mental are like two wings of a bird. They are complementary. Each of these depends on the other. In Kundalini Yoga, exercises occur automatically. Only those exercises that are really needed will occur during the process of cleansing.

D: All these exercises and meditation are just for the individual, for giving the divine feeling, etc. How does it affect society and the larger numbers of people? The difference between Eastern and Western philosophy is that the Eastern has always been for the individual. In the West, they have progress only because whatever they have done has been done for everyone.

G: When Shakti rises to the higher chakras, you will feel oneness in the true sense of the word for everyone around you. As a result of this you will not harm anyone. You will do things for other people because you feel like doing it, even much more than you do now. The power and basic creativity of the person increases, and as a result, your works will be much more effective. If many more people have this developed in them, then the level of tensions will be reduced.

D: How is it possible to carry the spirit of meditation with you every moment of the day?

G: When you breathe, you do not notice it. In the same way, in the later stages of meditation practice, you concentrate but you will not notice that you are concentrating. Until then you can continue to chant mentally.

D: Will bad habits go away with meditation or do you have to work on them yourself?

G: By practicing meditation regularly, bad habits will fall away automatically. In India, there are several cases where a robber became a saint through the practice of meditation. The same way you turn on the lights in a house to make the darkness vanish, good meditation makes the darkness and bad habits go away. There are many examples of people giving up smoking, drinking and other addictions once they began to meditate.

D: Does meditation burn up bad karma?

G: Meditation is like washing dirty clothes. In meditation we try to go to the real inner Self, and as we know more and more about it we tend to do good karma, which works against bad karma. It is not enough to do meditation only, but meditation does lead to doing good works. If one does meditation and then goes out and murders someone, the meditation would not help. There is a quality in real meditation that causes the desire to do bad things to drop away, slowly and automatically. Then, a person feels like doing good to others.

D: Why do I sometimes have such a clear, spiritual feeling, and why am I sometimes confused?

G: That is nothing new. That is natural. When you feel good, you have good meditations. When you don't feel good, you don't have good meditations. This will change with time. You will have more and more good meditations.

D: In meditation with you, the last two days I have had the most momentous experiences.

G: Yes. This is true for anybody who sits for at least five days. This is the holy sound of God. You will be filled with joy and energy through the sound. Many times while chanting I also go into meditation. No one will be without experiences. They must surrender to it.

D: I have been meditating for several years, but I do not feel any energy rising.

G: This takes time, it happens slowly. Do you have any guidance?

D: I was with another spiritual teacher for a while, but not now. I feel I need some guidance.

G: I will give you shaktipat. In no time you will start having more experiences. If you attend for four or five days you will feel the energy working in you.

D: I have been meditating for a long time, but I have never had the experiences I see other people having here.

G: This is the science of Kundalini Maha Yoga. In this science there are five different types of energy forces in the body: *prana, apana, samana, vyana* and *udana*. In Kundalini Maha Yoga they work together. When these forces work on the various chakras that are not yet open there will be some movements in the body. We call these kriyas. There are two types, physical and mental. The physical kriyas purify the body. During mental kriyas, imprints of the past births can come up and you may experience great joy. There are several different manifestations of joy: laughing, dancing, singing, jumping, vibrations in the body, or perspiration. These are all early stages of meditation. After reaching a certain level, one becomes steady and quiet.

D: What do kriyas cleanse?

G: Like a broom or a vacuum cleaner cleans a house, the kriyas cleanse the three bodies: physical, subtle and causal. The physical body has diseases and the potential for diseases; the others have other aspects of karma that need purification.

D: If an arm moves, or if you shake or feel something running up and down your spine, does this mean there is some blockage?

G: Your assumption is pretty good. It is the Kundalini working to clear an obstruction. For example, if there is a flood in a river, what will happen if there is a blockage? The water's force will build up there until it is cleared away. In a similar way, prana is working in the body.

D: When we get kriyas in a public meditation, in Guruji's presence, should we control them or let them go?

G: When possible, let the kriyas happen because they are what the Divine Energy has decided to do. But if they are noisy or disturbing, they should be controlled for the sake of others. If you block up flowing water, it may overflow, breaking the banks on both sides and causing damage. Energy is the same. If allowed to go on its own, it will go where it is supposed to go. In India, those with noisy kriyas sit in another room nearby. Those with quiet meditations sit with the main group.

D: Is pranayama considered noisy?

G: If it is too loud, yes.

D: If you have scratching or tickling sensations during meditation, should you go ahead and scratch?

G: It is better not to scratch. If it is uncomfortable, go ahead.

D: My arm was moving up and down while I was meditating tonight. Should I stop it? It seemed like it was getting pretty violent.

G: You should not stop it. Just let it happen. Were you doing it yourself or was it happening to you?

D: I don't know, I didn't start doing it purposely.

G: Then you do not have the right to stop it. Be a good boy and let the energy work. Don't get in the way.

D: Why do my hands, arms and legs get stiff during meditation?

G: Because the blood circulation is very slow and steady when you sit in meditation, the muscles get stiff. But that is only temporary. When you get up the stiffness will go away. Many times, yogis get as stiff as wood because of the slow circulation but it returns to normal automatically.

D: In Hatha Yoga, some asanas are more natural for me than others. Is it the same in meditation?

G: Hatha Yoga is only a preparation for meditation. Do meditation with the help of Guru and the awakened Kundalini. You will get those kriyas that you require. They happen naturally after the Kundalini is awakened. The Kundalini will do all the purification necessary for the body.

D: Is it good to do the kinds of meditation that are easiest for you?

G: You should try different things to find out which are suitable for you. All roads lead to the goal. Some people bicycle, some take an airplane. The choice depends on how fast you want to go. Also, it depends on your teacher.

D: Do certain kriyas have to do with certain chakras?

G: Yes. Even when you do not experience any kriyas physically, they may be occurring on the subtle or causal level. The specific kriyas that should take place, and for what purpose, is known only to the Shakti, but we may be able to understand when we are advanced enough.

D: Would you explain why kriyas occur in dreams?

G: In the same way that your body digests food and circulates blood while you are sleeping, the work of the Shakti goes on whatever you are doing. That is the importance of Kundalini Maha Yoga. Once the Shakti is awakened, She goes on working whether you want Her to or not.

D: Does one have to complete certain kriyas before going on to another stage?

G: Once the Kundalini energy is activated it is up to Her. She knows what kriyas are required. They come from this inner guidance. Even though you are treated for some sickness and get cured, you may get sick again. If you overcome one stage, you can go back again. If the kriyas are needed for purification, they will continue.

D: Sometimes I get very warm and sometimes I get cold during meditation. Is it the same kind of energy?

G: There are two nadis in the body related to the Sun and the Moon. When the Sun is working, you get hot. When the Moon is working, you become cold. It is not a difference in energy but in the channels it is taking.

D: My circulation seems off-balance. My right side is hot and my left side is cold. Is this from meditation?

G: Yes. One time in India, two people were each massaging one of my feet. One asked me why my foot was so hot and I said, "Maybe I have a high fever." The other asked me why my foot was so cold and I told him, "Maybe I'm about to die." So both started crying. Don't worry. It is a good sign.

D: Why is heat created in meditation?

G: When the Kundalini is awakened and active, the prana energy descends and the apana energy rises. They strike each other in the navel region and as a result heat is created all over the body. This is a cleansing process. The nadis get purified because of the generation of heat. Thus, these passages are cleared for the Kundalini to work through. The heat is actually generated prior to the upward movement of the Kundalini, just like the security guards clear a way when the President is coming so that he can move along quickly. Similarly, the prana and apana together work to clear a path for the Kundalini.

D: Is heat from meditation harmful?

G: If it is not controlled, it could be harmful. That is why you should drink milk with a little butter in it, or take coconut water or orange juice to control it. If the fire in a building is allowed to burn out of control, the whole building may burn up, so you should try to control it. But if you think the heat is some disease or that you have a fever and you start taking medicines, then again, you may damage yourself. The heat keeps decreasing as you progress and eventually you will reach a stage where you won't mind it. It will not be uncomfortable for you at all. You learn to live with it. There still may be periods where there is too much heat but you will be able to bear it.

D: During meditation sometimes I feel heat and pressure in my head. It is very uncomfortable and brings me out of meditation. My mind is no longer concentrated on one point. Is there anything I can do about it?

G: Take milk with butter in it and drink a lot of orange juice. If you still feel uncomfortable, you can massage almond oil on your head.

D: Is it true that the aroma of flowers will also keep the heat down?

G: Yes, it is true. Roses will do that.

D: Pressure builds up in my head during the day and it seems the only way to relieve it is to meditate. Meditation seems to disperse it more and more.

G: This is a good sign. The kriya has started in your body. If you cannot take the pressure, make it a habit to meditate daily. If you have not taken initiation, the effect will be only a temporary one, but after initiation it will be permanent.

D: What causes pressure in the head?

G: When prana flows upward sometimes you can feel pressure. When your capacity increases you will no longer feel it. It is like drinking beer. At first many people do not like it, but eventually you get used to it and develop a taste for it.

D: What does it mean when you feel cool water moving in your head?

G: This is an excellent experience. Heat is generated in the body. To cool your head, automatically, you experience a sensation of water.

D: I sometimes have a sense of power flooding my head. It is a beautiful feeling of pressure, like filling a balloon with something delightful. What is happening?

G: It could be called bliss. Cosmic bliss is higher. If you are eating a sweet dish you like, you feel about the same way.

D: On occasion, when I am meditating, forms come from the side to the center of my head and then they disappear. They have different colors. I don't understand what is happening.

G: When one is meditating, prana becomes one with apana. When you get a machine going there is a lot of activity. Similarly, when prana and apana unite, there is a lot of action and reaction with the five basic elements: earth, air, fire, water and space. These, mixed with your own samskaras, create the experiences you have in meditation.

D: Sometimes when meditating I get the feeling that two bodies want to come together but do not quite make it. I think I am in one, and something wants to break through. What does this mean?

G: All of us have three bodies: physical, subtle and causal. When meditating, these three bodies tend to become separated. Eventually you will experience this fully in meditation.

D: The separating or the coming together?

G: You feel this way now, but eventually you will feel it as a separation. The physical body is like a house. The subtle body, which takes the shape of the physical body, is like the electrical system. The causal body is composed of all past karmas. That body is in the akasha (sky).

D: When I meditate, my breath is really slow and even. All of a sudden there will be a feeling or sound in my chest, but it is not physical. My breath continues smoothly.

G: When the wind is blowing and passes through a narrow place, there will be sound. Similarly, if the passages of the vital forces are blocked by impurities, there may be sounds during meditation.

D: I would like to ask about the sounds in the ears. Why does one ear have a sound sometimes, while the other one has no sound? Sometimes I hear a high pitched sound like bells in my right ear.

G: All sounds that you hear internally are the sounds of God, especially the sounds you hear in the right ear. It is called the *Nada*, the sound of God that leads to liberation. Most of the sounds in the left ear are the sounds of Maya, and are binding. You are very lucky if you are only hearing them in the right ear.

D: Tonight I heard a high-pitched sound externally. It became greater until that sound was all there was. It was extremely electrical.

G: That is the *Omkara*, the cosmic sound. It has been there from the beginning of the universe. You can become one with that. The Kundalini is awakened by that sound and you ultimately reach oneness with God through it. Just as this electric light is not just for one person in the room but is for everyone, so it is with the holy sound of God. The yogi who has control of prana can create the holy sound. Even if you do not know the meaning of the sound, it can affect you. You do not have to know the meaning of fire for it to burn you.

D: When I hold my eyes a certain way when I meditate, I see a circle of light with a blue dot in it. What is it, and what should I do?

G: The light is the light of the soul and the spot is *bindu*, meaning a dot. There is a special branch of yoga you are going through by this initiation. You should just watch it. You do not have to do anything. You are not working towards that, it is coming by itself. Do not even have doubts whether it is your imagination or not. It is a very good experience.

D: I saw a light in meditation, and then I went through it. Is it all right to meditate this way?

G: There is a dawn before sunrise. At dawn you don't see the whole light yet, but soon there will be plenty of light. What you saw is the sign of sunrise.

D: When I meditate I see light and I find it hard to come out of meditation. Also, I don't have guidance from anyone.

G: You need guidance from someone familiar with this type of meditation. You are lucky to have such experiences. It is proof that your soul is pure and trying to grow further. There will be good progress on the spiritual path.

D: Sometimes when I am asleep I am awakened by a large, strong light in front of me. It makes me shake.

G: The light is your own and is not from outside. It is because you have done some good deeds in a previous life. This is the light of your soul and it is not separate from you. There are nine kinds of light of the soul. They are like fog, like smoke, like the Sun, like the Moon, like fire, like water, like electricity, like fireflies, and like crystals. Different people experience different kinds of light. Light is a sign of your progress, just as your coming here and meeting me is proof that I am here. If I am not here, you can come to this room and remember that I was here. In spiritual progress, the light means the same thing. It is a good sign of progress.

D: What is the significance of seeing a conch shell in meditation?

G: This is a very good indication. If you visualize the lotus, a beautiful baby, a white cow, an elephant or a white cobra, these are very good signs of spiritual progress. If you are going to undertake some work and meet any one of these objects, it is a very good omen of success in your task. All of these things are significant on both the physical and spiritual levels.

76

D: I saw the color green in meditation. Does this have a meaning?

G: Everything material is made of five elements: earth, air, fire, water and space. The colors you see depend on which elements are acting most on you. Earth is yellow, water is white, fire is red, air is green, and space is blue-black.

D: I had a Kundalini experience five years ago. It was fantastic. Nothing has been as good since. Is that the only time it will happen?

G: If you follow proper sadhana you will get experiences continually. You must have an accumulation of money in the bank before you can spend it. It is the same with the Kundalini energy.

D: Can you explain the power of visualization and how to develop it?

G: Meditation is the way. With the progress of the Kundalini Shakti you will attain various kinds of powers, including visualization.

D: How old should children be before being brought to meditation?

G: If it is just to meet me, any age at all. They may be brought to meditation itself if they are able to understand and be still.

D: My 10 year old daughter wants to come very badly.

G: Then bring her. In India, many small children meditate. They can have good experiences. When they are adults it will be easy for them to be on the spiritual path. Yogini, who is 6 years old and has had initiation, has told her mother to "Come and sit in meditation." There was a child of 6 or 7 in Denver. I asked her, "Do you wish to see your father?" (He was in Chicago). She said that she did, so I instructed her to meditate in the *puja* room. She went into a deep meditation. Afterwards, I asked her what she saw. She answered, "I saw some lights and someone sitting at a table." I told her mother to call the father, and she found that at that moment he was writing a letter home. Children are innocent. Their minds are very clear. If they are interested in meditation it is very good, so they should come.

D: Three times I have had the experience during meditation that I could wish anything and it would come to pass. What does this mean?

G: Once the Kundalini is awakened, any wish of the disciple is fulfilled, providing it is good, of course. For example, there was a disciple in India who wanted to rid his house of rats, so he wrote me asking for help. I told him to do a sankalpa before sitting in meditation and to pray to Mother Kundalini that the rats would not disturb him. He did this, and the rats stopped bothering him. Then, after a few days, he found that there were children outside bothering him. So again he did the same thing and the children stopped bothering him. If there is anything that is a hindrance to your spiritual progress, then just by wishing you can get things accomplished.

There is another example of a disciple in India who was very involved in politics. The opposition party got him charged with murder and took him to court, but he was actually innocent. He came to see me and to ask my advice. I told him, "Don't worry. Your Kundalini is awakened and She is taking care of you. I will help you also." I gave him a short mantra to recite. In a few days it so happened that the judge had to leave town because his mother fell sick. He took a month's leave and went off. Another judge came to replace him and as the proceedings were going on, it happened that the people talking against him started to forget things and to say things that were contradictory to their written statements. On that basis the judge dismissed the case, and the disciple was freed. So there is always protection. In the same way, the Kundalini is always protecting you, as well as trying to fulfill your wishes.

D: How important is it to remember what happens in meditation? Is there a way to try to remember?

G: You might be getting a significant message in your meditation, some event which might occur in the future or something regarding your spiritual progress. It is important that you remember it. You should do a sankalpa before meditation that you will remember it. Once you wake up, write it down right away.

D: I have heard that it is not good to talk about our experiences in meditation. Is that true?

G: If you are talking to someone who is also meditating, then it is all right. But if you talk to a stranger who would not understand, then it would not be appropriate. There could be a loss of energy.

D: Can a person attain self-realization without any visions or experiences of kriyas?

G: If you don't understand, maybe you won't recognize them. It is inevitable that you must go through certain experiences. You may not know you are going through a door but you must go through certain doors. Kriyas are neither necessary nor inevitable. They do not happen to everybody, but if any of your three bodies needs purification, then the kriya will happen. A healthy person needs no medicine but a sick person does. Some disciples have no kriyas but have good experiences.

Whenever one experiences great joy or bliss, this also manifests physically as crying or laughing. There are two kinds of kriyas. One is for purification, and one for the manifestation of joy. When we are talking, we gesture with our hands, even without noticing them. Similarly, when you experience things in meditation, you may not notice it.

SHAKTIPAT

D: Have you ever refused anyone that has asked for Shaktipat initiation?

G: I accept everyone. Only God can judge. You do not know who is good and who is bad in this world—only God knows. I work only to give. My work is to teach. I am God's agent. Rain falls everywhere. It doesn't just fall on the land or the rivers or the ocean. It falls everywhere. Rainfall is like bliss. My work is to distribute this God-given energy. Read the life of Jesus. All the people of a village wanted to kill a woman. They were throwing stones at her. Jesus came and asked, "Why are you stoning this lady?" They replied, "She is an adulteress." Jesus said to them, "Let he who is without sin cast the first stone," and sent them away.

Who knows who is a sinner and who is not? Only God knows. It is not my property. I am like a bank agent. All the property belongs to the company, not to the agent. The agent only manages it. He cannot refuse to give you your money on deposit whether you are a good person or a bad person. He cannot say, "I won't give you your money." If someone has a fever, he goes to a doctor. Why would you go to a doctor if you were healthy? If you have problems, difficulties, ignorance, fear or desire, you can go to church or to a saint. If you do not have such afflictions, then why would you go to a saint or to church? When you have the need, you go to a saint. His work is to give. He does not inquire whether you are a sinner or not. God's work is to benefit all people. God does not refuse anyone who goes to the church. So it is not my property. I am only the agent distributing it.

D: How do you explain Shaktipat besides transfer of energy?

G: The disciple is like a candle. The wick is ready. The wax is ready. All it needs is a match to light it. This is what initiation is. The guru is the fire, and all he has to do is light you up.

D: I see you have the picture of Christ on the altar. What relation is He to that analogy?

G: Every saint works for the welfare of mankind. Whether the saint is living or not, they actually are always helping. I have a high regard for Christ. That is why his picture is here, helping us now. There are many other saints who are not physically present but are helping us and guiding us at the astral level.

Christ was also a great yogi. Anyone that preaches "when someone strikes you on one cheek, you should turn the other cheek" has the idea of universality in him. He was a great believer in non-violence. He was a great saint and a great person. The healing that Christ performed by touch was Shaktipat. Energy in this sense is universal. It is a universal phenomenon. The sun is for everyone. Whenever a great upheaval takes place on earth, God incarnates Himself—He comes down. This belief is similar in both Hinduism and Christianity.

D: Does a fully realized guru have the ability to awaken the Kundalini of everyone? Does the energy automatically flow from one to the other?

G: A perfected yogi can awaken the Kundalini of anyone. The energy flow will be present anyway, but it is more intense when he directs it. Also, the results will depend on the recipient's openness. If one is not open, he may not receive the energy. When it is raining covered pots will not get any water, but the open ones will.

D: How do you know if you are ready to take initiation?

G: How do you know if you are hungry? God and the guru are willing to give. It is up to the person to receive it. He must desire it.

D: Initiation seems like something not to take lightly. Should one wait until they meet someone they know they should take initiation from, or does one take initiation from someone they think they should take initiation from?

G: It is all right to take initiation from a perfected guru, even if it is at the level of thinking. You can tell by the following signs if the yogi or guru is perfected or not: You experience your prana flowing upwards in his presence, your mind becomes calmer, you feel a great joy in his presence. Then, even if it is at the thinking level, the not-knowing level, it is right to take initiation. Once you experience any of these feelings, it is like sitting at a dining table with a meal before you when you are hungry. You do not start thinking and deciding, you just start eating. At that time you do not sit watching the food, wondering how much it cost and where it came from, whether it is good for you or contains poison. If you are hungry, you just start eating. Similarly, if you have some of the experiences I just described, and you desire it ardently, then you take it.

D: Is it necessary that you experience Shaktipat physically? I didn't feel anything physically. I just felt a lot of peace.

G: Shaktipat is experienced differently by everyone. The experience is according to their past karma and mind impressions, samskaras.

D: If one is following another spiritual path and asks you to perform Shaktipat, must he then give up that other path and follow yours?

G: If by following another path you are getting peace of mind and making progress, then I do not wish to confuse you. It is up to you to decide what to do. If you are going to one college and are not satisfied, you can change colleges. But that does not necessarily mean that you were not happy before. Rather, if you want more than what you were getting, you can take initiation.

D: Is it all right to do several types of spiritual practice at the same time, such as Buddhism or other types of yoga?

G: If you go to a shop to buy clothes, you choose a garment that you like. But you cannot go out wearing many clothes at once, no matter how many have appealed to you. In the same way, religion is for the enlightenment of the soul. When a certain path is right for you, you will know it and you should follow it.

D: If you receive Shaktipat from one guru, is it all right to receive it again from another guru?

G: If one doctor treats you but your disease is not cured, would you go to another doctor? If you are not satisfied and you think you need something more, then you can do it.

D: Can one have more than one guru?

G: Have you heard of Ramakrishna Paramahansa? He went to five different gurus when he felt a need.

D: If one guru has awakened the Kundalini, what is the point of taking other initiations?

G: If you have the experience that the Kundalini is awakened and moving upward, there is no need. If it is stuck, then it would be helpful to take initiation with another guru. It depends on one's own understanding of the problem. Suppose someone is earning $20,000 a year. If that is not enough, he may change jobs so that he can earn $40,000.

D: Can it actually hurt, however, if the Kundalini is moving? Can you damage your sadhana in any way?

G: In taking initiation from the right person, there is no question of damage. If the energy must be diverted in another direction, then the question of damage arises. Ramakrishna Paramahansa had the blessing of Ramani. He had visions of Shakti and was enjoying his own spiritual efforts. Then he went to another saint and he did the sadhana of Rama. Then he underwent Muslim guidance, then followed Hanuman. Once while living in Calcutta, a saint named Totapuri asked him if he was able to arrive at *Nirvikalpa samadhi*, which is pure bliss without thought.

Totapuri told Ramakrishna, "If you want to learn that, I will give you initiation." Ramakrishna said that he would go and ask the Mother Goddess. Totapuri was surprised and wanted to know who that mother was, the natural mother or another? He replied that it was the basic energy source behind all existence, that is his Mother. Totapuri said, "Yes then, go ask her." Ramakrishna asked the Goddess if he should get help to achieve samadhi, and the Mother gave her permission. Ramakrishna went to Totapuri, took initiation, and had the experience of Nirvikalpa samadhi for three days and nights continuously. It was a big surprise to Totapuri also. Totapuri had to chant "Hari Om" in his ears to bring him back to this level of consciousness. Does this answer your question?

D: Does a disciple really have a choice in the matter? I felt that I was swept along without having to choose.

G: What is working is past karma. Whether you desire it or not, you are swept into it. If someone's karma is not "ripe enough," they will sometimes sit with the guru but not take initiation.

D: In preparation for initiation, which center should we concentrate on most, the crown chakra or the third eye center?

G: When you are hungry, do you find that you are satisfied before eating or after eating? Real progress starts after initiation. Concentrate your attention on the third eye and follow your breath.

D: What is the relationship between Kundalini, Shaktipat and kriya movements?

G: Kundalini is the car, Shaktipat is the driver, and kriyas are the motion of the car.

D: Since Shaktipat I am hungry all the time. Do I eat too much? Should I fast?

G: If you are hungry in the months after Shaktipat, it is the Kundalini work-ing. You should not fast. To do so could be damaging. One disciple was so hungry; he was eating enough for eight men. He asked me what he could do. I told him to eat outside instead of with the others inside, so that they wouldn't be surprised. He did so for three months. After some time this problem will level out.

D: I find that I am not so hungry after Shaktipat. Is it all right to fast in that case?

G: That is all right. Fasting is good for the mind if one is not hungry. In India we fast two times a month for one day. We take only liquids.

D: After Shaktipat, in some people there is no noticeable change in tem-perament. Why is this?

G: Those people who have good past karma are affected much sooner. Those who need a lot of cleansing take a little longer. The process is started in either case. If a doctor gives the same medicine to two differ-ent patients, one may get better sooner than the other, depending on the damage done to the body and what needs to be cured. The person with less damage will show signs of getting better much sooner.

D: Do we learn this path instantaneously at the moment of Shaktipat, or do we learn by coming here and listening to questions and answers?

G: Sitting, meditating and feeling peaceful is good, but unless you are initi-ated, it may be like going to a drama. When you go home, you will forget about it. After initiation, a permanent link is established between you and the guru. If the wind splashes water on the land surrounding a lake, it is helpful. But it is not as helpful as having a canal that system-atically irrigates the land. Initiation is like irrigation.

D: After Shaktipat, does spiritual progress depend on the purification of the mind and body?

G: Once you have been initiated, the Shakti takes over and does the necessary purification. Your job is to meditate regularly and follow the instructions of the guru. After initiation, the guru has provided you with a car, filled it with gas, taught you how to drive and shown you the road. All you have to do is drive the car. If you do not drive, you will be sitting in the same spot.

D: To receive initiation, must one accept you as a guru?

G: Whatever benefit you have to gain is for yourself. If you want to take initiation and accept me as your guru, you are going to have the maximum gain. If you take the initiation and do not accept me as your guru, you will gain a certain amount but not the maximum. You have nothing to lose and everything to gain. If you are learning from a college professor but start criticizing him and arguing with him, how is he going to teach you? If you accept what he teaches and have some faith in him, then you are going to benefit. You are taking the initiation for your benefit, not for the guru's. A guru is here only to give. You are the one who has to receive. In the scriptures, a saint has written a poem that says, "God and guru are both standing in front of me. Who should I bow down to first, God or guru? It is because of the guru that I have realized God. It is by the guru's guidance and grace that I have finally merged with God. God was always there but I never realized it. It has been by the guru's grace that I have come to realize it. So I should bow down to the guru first. The servant of God is greater than God, because God is always there even though I never saw Him. It was the servant of God that helped me to see God, so he is greater than God." So your faith and devotion to a guru is for your welfare, not for anyone else's.

I want to give an example of what the guru does. Tulasidas was a great saint. In India, the yogis usually go around with bare feet. I also walked around India for 20 years without shoes in every type of weather, extremely hot or in the snow and rain. This is a story about Saint Tulasidas.

He was doing some austerities and his guru came by. "By the grace of that guru who has led me to God, I bow to that guru's feet. Just as sunlight removes darkness, so by the grace of my guru the darkness has been eliminated from my mind. It is very difficult to get the Kundalini awakened, but by guru's grace, it becomes very easy." He removed the sand clinging to the feet of his guru, collected it and put in a plate and prayed to his guru. Saint Tulasidas said, "This sand is precious to me, even like sand from the feet of God. This sand is love-giving. This sand is peace-giving. I bow down to it. This sand is so pure that, just as medicines can cure diseases, this sand will give me liberation from the miseries of this world."

It is said in the scriptures that Lord Shankara used to meditate in the graveyards because when you meditate in such places you develop a very strong sense of detachment, knowing that we are all going to die one day. In India, we cremate the bodies of the dead. When Lord Shankara was meditating, the sand used to fly around and stick to his body. The devotees would collect the sand and keep it in their house because it is considered very pure and peace giving. It caused good things to happen in the house.

Saint Tulasidas said, "The sand from the feet of my guru belongs to the same category as that sand from Lord Shiva's body, which is so pure. The sand from the feet of my guru is so pure that as sand can polish the surface of a mirror, so this sand can remove the darkness of my mind. The nails on the feet of my guru shine like pearls. By meditating on them, I can have divine visions and become purer. By applying the sand to my eyes and forehead, my problems are removed. Just as when the Sun comes up and removes all darkness, so by the grace of my guru, all negative qualities of my mind are eliminated." By having devotion to the feet of a guru, you can gain knowledge of God. By the grace of the guru, things of the worldly life that seem impossible become very easy. You start gaining knowledge of things that are normally invisible to you, knowledge of things of the universe. Once the Kundalini is awakened and reaches the crown chakra, the Sahasrara, you receive knowledge of everything that exists. Many things which modern science has discovered with the help of instruments like microscopes and telescopes, the yogis of India described in great detail thousands of years ago through visions in meditation.

If a person does not know what the Kundalini is, then it may be difficult. By the grace of a perfected guru, if he has control over prana and can awaken the Kundalini, then there is no problem. The Kundalini is a source of happiness, but if people do not know how to control Her they may have some difficulties. So I advise them to go to a perfected guru. Then everything will be all right.

THE GURU

D: Does one need a guru to achieve perfection?

G: If you want to get a college degree, do you get it by sitting at home? A seed needs to be sown in the ground in order to grow. It needs earth, water, manure and someone to take care of it. If a seed disregards all that and says, "I am going to sit here and try to grow," it is not going to work. In the same way, you need some guidance.

D: There have been exceptions, though, of people who have been God-realized without having a physical guru.

G: Those are very rare. Those people have already achieved certain goals in previous births, and have come back to help other people. Their mind impressions have already been purified in other lives, and they have reached the highest goal. They return only to help others, not to realize themselves. You cannot attain much knowledge on your own. It will take you many times longer. The guru is there to guide and help you.

D: Does everyone need a guru?

G: A guru is a teacher. You have always needed teachers, like when you were a child in school. On the spiritual path, too, everyone needs a teacher. You need light to get out of darkness. A guru brings that light. The laborers who break stones do not like that hard work but they must do it to attain their goal. To attain what you want you must go through it. Everyone is born with fear. Do not be afraid. You cannot learn to swim without going in the water. Everyone is afraid at first. The cause of fear is not having any guidance. If you are ill, you go to a doctor to get medicine. On the spiritual path, you also need guidance, otherwise progress may stop. If you do not have guidance, you do not know how to be protected. What you experience as fear is Maya, illusion. All must overcome it.

D: Is there a certain guru for every person?

G: You can go on looking until you find peace. You may go to a college and not be happy, so you go to another one. If you are not happy with a particular guru, you can go on looking. Until you are satisfied you will look for another one. There are many persons who could be your guru, but you should stick to the one from whom you get the light.

D: I have heard that a person might meet many gurus before deciding there was one particular one who was a channel to God for him.

G: It is not always so, but at times it may be like that, depending on karma. Your karma might say that there is one particular guru for you but not necessarily.

D: How do you go about finding a guru?

G: When your inner urge is really strong, a guru will appear. Right now you are receiving guidance because you are here.

D: What are the characteristics of a true guru?

G: Various characteristics have been mentioned in the scriptures. If you see these in another person, then he or she might be a true guru. When a real desire occurs in your heart to find a real guru, then God presents one to you. When you go near a true guru, you get an upward feeling, your energy flows upward. The impure thoughts in your mind calm down and are replaced by pure ones. When you sit near such a guru, you feel pleasure and you don't want to get up and leave his or her presence. You feel peace of mind. You feel that the guru does not have any selfish interests.

D: I have been trained in Kundalini Yoga and was exposed to a guru for three years in an ashram, but my guru died. Now I am questioning. It does not seem right and natural. Sometimes in meditation things happen but I wonder if it is real experiences or just my imagination.

G: If you have a question about whether it is right or not, then it is not. That is why you are not satisfied. Maybe you need proper guidance. Sometimes you sit down to a meal and eat but are not satisfied. The same is true here.

D: What is it that determines the ripeness of the disciple for receiving the guru's grace? What determines the disciple's ability to grow spiritually?

G: Obedience to the guru. For example, one guru had two disciples. One was smart and clever, and the other was innocent and simple. After a day of work, the two disciples were massaging his legs. He said to the smart one, "Go and see if the rain has stopped." It had been raining since the day before, and as the house was made of weak material, it was necessary to take precautions that the house did not collapse. The smart disciple said, "Gurudev, the rain has stopped." The guru replied, "You didn't go out to check it. How do you know it has stopped?" The smart disciple said, "Look at the cat. She has come in from outside and she is dry." But the guru said, "The cat doesn't go outside. She stays inside." The smart disciple said, "No. She goes out each day at this time, and the fact that she is dry proves that there is no more rain."

Then the guru said to the smart disciple, "Then the oil lamps are pointlessly burning outside. Go put them out so there is no wastage." The smart disciple replied, "Gurudev, there is no need for us to go turn them off because once we close our eyes we won't be able to see them." Then the guru told him, "Then go and close the door of the compound so no one will enter."

The smart disciple replied, "Gurudev, I did two of the three things you asked me. Why don't you do this third thing?" The smart disciple was asked to sit to one side. The guru told him, "Now you can go home. You are not prepared for further training."

Now it was the turn of the innocent disciple. He used to cook for the guru. One day, half an hour after lunch, the guru said, "Why not cook for me? I am hungry." He cooked again and he brought it to Gurudev. Then Gurudev told him, "This is no good, why don't you cook something else?"

He cooked again. Then the guru told him, "Why don't you give this food to the dog. I am not hungry and I don't want to eat." So it was given to the dog.

The next day the guru was reading outside in the sun. He told his disciple, "Why don't you go and get a lamp for me, I can't see. There is not enough light." So he went inside and brought the lamp. When the disciple took the lamp to the guru, he blew it out. When night came and the lamp was burning again, the guru told his disciple, "Please turn it out. I want to read in the dark." So he blew it out.

At that time the guru blessed him with his hand on his forehead and said, "You will have knowledge of the truth," and he attained all knowledge with the touch of his guru. If the feeling between the guru and the disciple is like this, all knowledge can flow to the disciple.

D: If, when the guru asks us to do something, we should do it, what about our own mental feelings concerning what we should do? Should we forget our own set of do's and don'ts?

G: The things you create with your own mental views are likely to be misleading. Your mind may be playing tricks on you, whereas the guru can lead you on the right path. It is best to follow the guru. However, you can still have your own feelings and concerns and use your intellect.

D: What does it mean to surrender to the guru?

G: Surrender means that you have firm faith and devotion to him and for the subject that he is teaching. Only under those conditions can he impart full knowledge to you. When you are fully receptive he will not hide anything from you. He will teach everything freely. It is just like going to college. If you are open and have respect for your subject and the teachers, then you can learn and progress. If you are resistant and do not agree with what your teachers are saying, then you cannot learn very much. It is mainly firm faith and devotion that will help you. Surrendering also means that you become like a child. As long as you were a baby, your mother took care of you. She fed you when you were hungry and kept you warm. Once you grew up, then you took care of yourself. Similarly, if you become like a child, then the guru can take care of you. By surrendering to him and accepting what he has to say, you can progress very rapidly.

Krishna's main disciple was Arjuna. One day there was a pigeon nearby and Krishna said to Arjuna, "What do you see?" He replied, "I see a pigeon". Krishna said, "No, I think it is a peacock." Arjuna replied, "Yes, my Lord, it is a peacock." Then Krishna said, "No, I think it is a swallow." Arjuna answered, "Yes, my Lord, it is a swallow." Then Krishna said, "No, I think it is a cow." And Arjuna answered, "Yes, it is a cow." Krishna asked, "Why do you just accept what I say? Why don't you use your own intelligence?" He answered, "My intelligence is limited. You being the Lord, your intelligence is limitless, so whatever you say is acceptable to me." That is being absorbed. Surrender means obedience to the guru.

D: What should you do if you have doubts?

G: That is just your ego playing. It is in your hands to destroy it. When you feel a lack of peace within yourself, you know you are lacking something. That is why you go to someone else for knowledge. As long as you are in that state, you should just forget your ego and surrender. If you can allow yourself to become like a child again you will progress from then on.

When you go to school, you do not learn everything in one day. You must practice. If you assume that you know everything you will not learn. It is best to just surrender. A student who goes to college doesn't know if he will succeed, but he begins with the faith that he will be successful. Similarly, you should have faith that you will be successful. Just keep working and you will start to have experiences that will increase your faith and devotion. That is why some people have kriyas in their bodies. It is a sign of the awakened Kundalini so they will stick to the path and progress. These experiences are not the ultimate goal; they are a means to the goal.

D: Can a guru transmit his wisdom to someone who is a complete skeptic?

G: It is enough to be a human being and searching. Vivekananda was a skeptic. He was searching for someone that claimed to see God. When he found one, he believed. So it can happen. A guru means one who leads from darkness to light. Skepticism is darkness.

D: What does the guru get from the disciple?

G: A guru is a giver, not a taker. It is the disciple who is the taker. The disciple can give dedication and a sense of surrender. When that is complete then he will get maximum benefit. The rains come from the sky, but the farmer must keep his fields ready with plowing and planting. If he does not do so, he will have no benefit when the rains come. You must keep your fields ready through dedication and surrender.

D: Is the guru-disciple relationship a friendly relationship, a father-son relationship, or how should the disciple regard the guru?

G: There is no withdrawal of any kind of feeling with a guru. In the words of the *Guru Arati* it is said:

Tvam Eva Mata,	You are my mother,
Cha Pita Tvam Eva,	You are my father,
Tvam Eva Bandush,	You are my brother,
Cha Sakha Tvam Eva,	You are my friend,

Tvam Eva Vidya,	You are knowledge,
Dravinam Tvam Eva,	You are wealth,
Tvam Eva Sarvam,	You are my everything,
Mama Deva Deva.	My God of Gods.

So it includes all relationships. Because you can have the feelings of all these relationships in one person, he can finally take you to liberation.

D: To help us understand, I would like to ask what Guruji did with his teacher?

G: To be respectful to the teacher, not to hurt his feelings, to obey him by following instructions very strictly, to have reverence for the knowledge he is giving, all these things are necessary. The guru does not desire it. It is for the disciple that it is necessary. For the benefit of the disciple, it is necessary that they bow and express their feelings.

D: Could you clarify some of the reasons for showing respect to the guru in these ways?

G: When you have that respect and that feeling for the guru, that manifests itself in forms of action. It purifies your mind and body. It is also true that you get energy from touching the guru's feet. This helps the disciple overcome his ego.

D: What kind of relationship did you have with your guru?

G: The worship that you do of the guru is not of his physical body but of the guru energy that is flowing from God. The supreme guru is God Himself. So you are worshipping that energy that is flowing through him to you. There is space outside and there is space that is confined by this building, but both spaces are related directly. In the same way the guru-energy of God, which is all pervading, is one and the same connected space.

D: In the traditional relationship of devotee and teacher, the devotee needs guidance from time to time for his spiritual progress. If the guru goes to another city, what chance is there for guidance?

G: The relationship between guru and disciple is the supreme relationship in human existence, even superior to that between mother and child. The mother only gives physical birth, but the guru leads you onto the path to liberation. If he is perfected, the guru need not be physically present. He can give you guidance from anywhere. Take Shri Aurobindo and Mataji for example. Even after they left their physical bodies, they continue to guide their disciples on a subtle level, both mentally and spiritually. So physical presence is not so important. It is the perfection of the guru and the relationship of guru and disciple that matters. Then physical limits are transcended. There are many yogi-gurus who have left the physical body and still guide their disciples.

When you become initiated, an astral bond is formed with the guru and his physical presence is no longer necessary. I can guide you from a distance. Right now, I am guiding many people in India while I am here in the United States. Often a guru can make contact with the soul of people around him, as well as their questions, for the Atman is one and the same. So he can make connections with people here and in India.

D: In a dream, Guruji tapped me on the head. I both heard it and felt it. What does that mean?

G: This is a blessing; you will have it again but do not desire it consciously. Wish for it; then forget it. If you desire their presence, yogis will come because of your desire but they prefer to come on their own. However, if you pray for me, I will definitely be there.

D: Can you see our obstructions clairvoyantly and remove them?

G: If I point my mind towards that, yes.

D: Do you hear what I am saying without words?

G: Only if I choose to do so.

D: Aside from the meditation and mantra we were taught, is it possible to do more spiritual work, such as *anusthan* and austerities, without the physical presence of the guru to guide us?

G: In any case where you want to do sadhana other than what your guru has recommended, it is essential to have his guidance, not necessarily his physical presence.

D: Does that mean that we should be in touch by letter or telephone?

G: Yes. In Sanskrit for example, words often have double meanings. It would be possible to confuse one word in a sentence and change the meaning from "Protect this wife" to "Eat up this wife." So you need detailed instructions on mantras, etc.

D: Before I knew anything about gurus or Indians, I saw a beautiful face in meditation. The next day, a friend gave me Paramahansa Yogananda's book and the same face was on the cover. I wonder if I had been receiving guidance.

G: There are many yogis who are working like this from other planes. For example, there was a person in Attleborough who had a similar experience of seeing an Indian face. Shortly afterwards, an Indian friend showed her a number of photos and when she came to my photo, she recognized the face she had seen. Another example of this is a lady who had read Yogananda's book and said, "He is dead but I want a guru; what should I do?" So she prayed. The very next day, someone gave her a notice about our programs. She went to one, later became initiated, and is now making very good progress.

D: If a guru of another path appears in a dream, does that mean something?

G: It is we who think of different paths. For the gurus, it is one and the same. They are always giving blessings to help people reach God. Regardless of what path a person may be following, they can get visions of gurus from other traditions. That just indicates that they are receiving a blessing from that guru.

D: Do you believe that Jesus Christ is the disembodied guru for Westerners?

G: All people who have achieved realization are the same. There is not one for Westerners and another for Easterners. Ram, Buddha, Krishna, Jesus Christ—they are all the same.

D: What can his disciples do to make Guruji happy?

G: Do your sadhana and attain realization. That is my greatest joy. In one scripture, it says that one goes through eighty-four hundred thousand lives, and that one who attains liberation is spared the pains of so many births. There is no greater joy.

SADHANA AND THE SPIRITUAL PATH

D: What is the quickest and easiest way to Self-realization?

G: Know yourself. It's very simple—just know yourself.

D: But there is *Raja, Bhakti, Jnana, Karma* and many other forms of yoga. Which is best?

G: Whichever you feel is suitable for you, go after that one. They all lead to the same goal. Which is faster depends on you. Some people like sweet food, some sour, hot or bland. The basic thing is to feel content— no longer hungry. Whatever suits you is the best for you.

D: Is there a distinction between God-realization and Self-realization?

G: Self-realization comes first. That means to understand and feel what one's own Self is. Once you understand your own real Self, it is not difficult to understand about God. First, you must know what you are yourself. Without that, you cannot understand what God is. Once you experience your own Self, you will know that there is no difference between you and God. You will experience the fact that God's Shakti is all pervading. It is in everyone. Until you feel that they are not two different things, the realization has not come to you. Knowing that you and God are one is God-realization.

D: If God is everywhere, why don't we know him?

G: Between God and us is the wall of Maya. You cannot see him through the wall, so you do not see God. Ram, Sita and Lakshman are walking in the jungle. Ram is God, Sita is Maya and Lakshman is like the individual living being. Because Sita is in between, Lakshman cannot see Ram. In the same way, Maya separates the individual from God. To eliminate this obstruction we do sadhana—chanting, meditation—and once it is eliminated, the realization is there.

D: Do you mean to say that the individual soul is one of the illusions of Maya?

G: No. Maya is like a curtain between the soul and God. The soul is not an illusion and is not the same as Maya. By meditation, we remove the curtain and the individual merges with God. If you have water in a vessel and you throw it into the ocean, it becomes one with the ocean. There is no difference then.

D: Don't some yogis say that to externalize a concept of God is to weaken the direction one is taking since the object is to internalize?

G: If you say you want to become one with God, you are at the stage where you are two. That implies you need him to be outside. That is only a means for you to find the link, for you to find the oneness. Until you do, externalizing is natural. After that, you internalize. For example, you want to reach a city 100 miles away. On the road you see milestones. When you reach the last stone, you are not yet in the city but you have reached the city. It is externalized as the last milestone.

Another example: When you construct a building, you install scaffolding that comes down once the building is complete. All types of sadhana are instruments for reaching the final goal. They are not the goal itself, yet you cannot do without them.

D: Is it safe to assume that sadhana means living in the best way possible?

G: The basic question is, what is the right kind of life? Perhaps stealing? (Laughter) For some, devotion is the right life. So this is the first question. For guidance in this, perhaps a guru is needed. Once you know your correct path, you will know what is right and what is wrong.

D: What can I do to make life less painful?

G: Once you realize your own true identity, what is inside, your real Self, all such questions will be answered. To do this you need meditation.

Through this inner path the miseries of the world end. When you see the answer to the question "Who am I?" all problems are solved.

D: What is the purpose of practicing austerities?

G: To learn some new skill you have to keep trying. In the same way we study to attain a degree, we have to work to remove the effects of our bad karma, our harmful past actions. So, we do austerities to purify our bodies and minds.

D: Like what?

G: There are many kinds. If you do japa (repeat mantras) for 12 hours you do not have time for other kinds of work. That is all right.

D: Some say that unless you offer your work to some particular deity, it is valueless. Must it be offered to some particular personal aspect, or can it be offered just to God?

G: Yes. That is all right. You can offer it to the Lord who is all pervading, or to the Shakti.

D: Once the Kundalini has been awakened, can it go back to sleep again?

G: If awakened through Shaktipat, it never goes back to sleep again, but progress can be slowed if sadhana is neglected. If you are flying from L.A. to New York but the plane stops over in Chicago, the trip becomes much longer. If the Kundalini was awakened spontaneously, it is possible for it to become dormant again.

D: Should the "Om Ram" mantra be said 24 hours a day, only when you think of it, or at set times?

G: You can do it mentally 24 hours a day. Yogis estimate that one takes 21,600 breaths in one day. If your mind is one-pointed, you can do one mantra with each breath. When that becomes part of your system, it can go on for 24 hours as simply and naturally as your breath.

The poet Kabir says, "You have lost your life doing japa with your hand without putting your mind into it. Now is the time to give up the mala and do it in your mind." Some people do malas but let their minds wander all around. That is useless. If the japa becomes part of your breath, that is best. This is not to say that you should give up doing malas, but to emphasize the need to keep your mind on it.

D: Is it all right to do other mantras one might like—such as "Jesus Christ have mercy on me" or "Om Namah Shivaya"?

G: The different dishes in a meal have different purposes. So do different mantras. To do one particular mantra, especially the one given by your guru, is the best. The Bhuta Shuddhi mantra is for the purification of the physical, subtle and causal bodies so that meditation will be unobstructed. If you want to paint a wall, you clean it first. Similarly, if the body is pure meditation will be perfect. Do the Bhuta Shuddhi mantra three times before meditation. It will help.

D: Is it important to say the Sanskrit words of a mantra, or is saying it in English all right?

G: In a machine the parts are organized in a particular way so the mechanism can operate. Similarly, the sounds of a mantra are organized so as to give a specific effect. A prayer is all right in English, but a mantra is a mantra.

D: Should one visualize seed syllables while doing a mantra? Is that part of the technique?

G: This is one technique. You may do it if you like. But this visualization technique is more difficult than concentrating on the breath. If you are trying to dig a well, it is better to make one deep hole than to make shallow holes all over. If you are building a house, it is better to make one foundation than to start several.

D: Does it help to know that different colors come from different mantras?

G: That knowledge may be helpful but it is unnecessary. The mantras work without it. Suppose you are eating a sweet. Even if you don't know who made it or how it was made, you will enjoy it anyway.

D: Why are there 108 beads in a mala?

G: One hundred is a complete number signifying God. Anything completed is never exhausted. Then there are eight types of Maya: earth, water, fire, air, space, mind, intellect and ego. These exist between God and the individual living being.

If you want to see an important man, you have to get by his secretary first. Otherwise you might try for six months and never get an appointment. But if the secretary likes you, she will find a way to get you in, even if there is a big crowd waiting at the door. She just takes you in the back way. Similarly, if Maya Shakti is favorable to us She lets us see God, but not otherwise.

Many rich people have dogs to guard their houses. To get by them you must get the owner to let you in, or you must somehow control the dog with food or some other means. Similarly, if Maya Shakti does not want you to meet God, She will not allow it.

So the remaining eight beads of the mala are the beads of Maya. The one doing japa with the mala is the jiva—the individual living being. Eight of the beads are for Maya. One hundred are completion, God. So after passing through the eight, you go on to the hundred without problems. We must cross over Maya first. That is the meaning of the 108 beads of the mala.

D: Is japa beneficial even if my Kundalini is not awakened?

G: You may do as much japa as you wish, but until the door to the Sushumna is open the japa is not fruitful. If you have a basket full of fruit and candy and just look at them you will be unsatisfied. If you eat them you will be satisfied. If the Sushumna is open all forms of sadhana will be fruitful. Even if you eat a small piece of fruit there will be some satisfaction.

D: How can we speed up our progress?

G: Keep doing the Bhuta Shuddhi mantra, one mala a day, for 40 days and then leave off for awhile. Do japa in the mind constantly. Do your work with your hands and do japa in your mind.

D: During your early years of sadhana, did you ever feel loneliness even when feeling bliss?

G: Yes, I did at first. But then the mountains, rivers, streams—everything— became my own.

D: Is loneliness necessarily part of the spiritual path, something one has to go through?

G: It helps spiritual progress and makes it faster. If you are doing sadhana at home and think, "I'd like to go visit my friend," you will. In the mountains alone desires come, but then vanish. Soon being alone becomes a habit.

D: Because the desires can't be fulfilled?

G: When your basic purpose is spiritual attainment, desires are passing phases. Later, it becomes your nature not to desire things, to be one-pointed on the spiritual path.

D: How much should we isolate ourselves?

G: That is up to the individual, like how much you eat or how much you exercise. For some, even a lonely place is crowded. Others need only close their eyes in a crowded place to be alone. There is no specific prescription that is good for everyone. In my case, whether I am in a plane, a car, a living room, or some lonely place, the same high state is possible. One develops the habit of being always surrounded by solitude.

D: After you were awakened on the mountain, was there a time when your feelings kept on changing, like being full and then not having it?

G: Nobody stays in the same mental state all the time. If I had remained fixed in the same mental state I was in just after receiving Shaktipat from my guru, I would not be alive now to be with you.

D: What does it mean when the worshipful attitude phase leaves?

G: The jiva, the individual being, is very unstable. That is why you go through fluctuations. Gradually you will become stable and nothing will diminish. The jiva has five qualities: joy, sorrow, knowledge, ignorance and evil. Sometimes we are happy, sometimes sad. By being patient, we finally reach a stable stage. The jiva is part of God but once separated, like the individual rays separate from the Sun, it forgets, becomes ignorant and entangled in Maya. The jiva is dependent on Maya, not independent like God. It goes through these fluctuations as long as it is unrealized, but once it realizes its identity it becomes stable and merges with God. That is why you have to do sadhana to reach God.

D: How can I develop one-pointedness?

G: There is no magic in it. It requires practice like anything else. When you first went to school you knew nothing about writing. You tried to write "a" and did it a little differently each time until finally you learned. It requires effort.

D: So the spiritual path is a struggle?

G: When you try to learn something to please others — your father, for instance — there is struggle. Learning is for you. When you do it that way, it is not struggle but enjoyment.

D: How do you know that you are reaching a higher level of consciousness?

G: When you are eating, how do you know you are full? It is a matter of experience and cannot be told in words. You don't worry about it. You eat until you are satisfied.

D: People say that on the spiritual path one may mistake some lesser place for the final goal. How do you know that you are there?

G: When you go into a foreign country, you know it. When I came to America, I had a general idea about it, so when I arrived I knew it. The final stage of the spiritual path is no more desire, no more sorrow. When you have it, you will know it.

D: Yet I have heard that some yogis make a mistake and take their bliss for the final place, and do not recognize their error until death.

G: After he has reached the final stage, the yogi controls any birth he may take. They take birth only when, and if, they wish to. If they cannot do that, they are not at the final stage.

D: How can we protect ourselves from the many terrible experiences in the world without ruining our spiritual growth?

G: You have to learn to become indifferent to the world, to whatever may be happening around you. Jesus had to pass through terrible experiences, but even when he was crucified he did not react with anger. He blessed those who crucified him and the world worshipped him. Because Jesus adhered to his principles and because of his good heart, those who killed him repented afterwards.

D: Sometimes I am overcome with anger. How can I change this to love?

G: Where there is a fire, you must use water to cool it. Even though a mother may be angry with her child for crying out in need, she goes to it with love, forgetting her anger. You will observe that when you get angry, you become hot physically and your voice gets louder. First, lower your voice and start thinking about why you got angry and what will happen if you act on your anger. Keep thinking. Once you become the observer of your actions, you will start to cool off. Postpone action when you are angry, and your anger will dissipate.

D: I have a big problem with my ego.

G: Merge your will with the will of God, and He will melt your individual ego.

D: How?

G: You have to train yourself. You must continually remind yourself that in this world one cannot do anything by oneself. If the situation is right for it you can act, but not otherwise. Napoleon said there was no such word as "impossible" in his vocabulary, but at Waterloo he had to accept a higher truth. Your actions are not yours but God's. When you recognize that fully, your ego will merge with Him.

D: Will you distinguish mind and ego?

G: Mind, intellect and ego—all three are needed to accomplish anything. Suppose you see and hear an apple fall from a tree. The information about the apple falling enters through the eyes and ears to the brain that supports the mind. The intellect analyzes, thinks about the information and informs the ego that there is something worth having. Then the Self says "yes" to the ego, which commands the intellect, which directs the mind and nervous system to start walking towards the apple. Everything has a sequence but it operates so fast that we cannot separate out the parts in action. This process takes place in each good or bad action, whether or not to act is the choice of the Self. If, after this process of gathering information, the Self says not to act on it, nothing will happen and the brain will not order the hands and feet to get the apple.

Suppose you have a revolver. Unless you pull the trigger, it will not fire even if you wish to shoot someone. Although the desire exists, if you don't act on it, nothing will take place. The mind is like a horse, and the Self like the person who rides it. You have the reins in your hand and the power to control it. If you just let the horse go where it desires, it may take you anywhere, even into a ditch or a stream. So always keep the reins in your hand and guide the horse. Keep your Self in control and don't let the mind run away with you.

D: Is the will a function of the causal body?

G: A certain portion of will is conditioned by the samskaras of the causal body. Then the new karmas that you are doing add to the causal body that is there already. The cycle of existence comes from these three things: karma from the past, the fruits of this karma, and the new karma you create while undergoing the results of the old karma. This accumulated karma is the causal body. If you do whatever you do without attachment, the actions do not create new karma. The actions still have their consequences in the Maya of the world, but they do not bind and limit what you are.

D: Sometimes it seems that the ego and the intellect gang up on the Self.

G: That is the weakness of the Self at that stage. It listens to other things and can be short-circuited. Yogis say you should become independent, not the slave of the mind but its controller. You will see that once the Self becomes strong, nothing can prevail against it. Meditation teaches you that—how the Self can become independent and strong. No matter what your mind tells you, if you are strong you will not allow improper action. Although your ego and mind want you to quarrel with someone, if you do not act on that, no quarrel will take place.

D: Do we have free will, or is life like a book where we act out what is written?

G: First of all, in our life there are three basic factors determining our fate: (1) The accumulated karma of innumerable births, (2) the karma that has taken effect already in this lifetime forming our bodies and personalities, and (3) what we work for, our own efforts. Secondly, in everything that happens to us there are three contributing factors: (1) our own will, (2) the will of others and (3) the will of God. What happens to us is a combination of these. What God wills always happens. What we will, and what others will, may or may not happen.

For example, some years ago, Hitler was successful for awhile through a combination of his own will and the will of others. Then when God willed, he vanished from the scene. On the other hand, the work of Jesus was a combination of his will, the will of others and the will of God so it is important even 2,000 years later.

D: Hitler caused millions of people to die. Are you saying that was against the will of God?

G: The fact that he was unsuccessful in the end shows that his work was not the will of God. At this stage in your development, the puzzle is whether things happen because of your will or God's. When you reach the stage where you see that everything that happens occurs by God's will, you will no longer have this question. Acceptance of this fact is not a matter of intellectual judgment. You may challenge it saying, "I'll accept that if this building falls on me this instant." But even if it does not fall, that does not prove that things don't happen according to God's will.

D: How do I know God's will?

G: When, through your own purification and spiritual practice, you get nearer to God, you will know within yourself what God wishes.

D: Is it possible to reach the stage where God's will is our will, and God's thoughts are our thoughts?

G: This is a purpose of the spiritual path.

D: In *Message to Disciples* you seem to recommend celibacy until realization, but in the instructions for Shaktipat you say to remain celibate from one to three months, or as the situation requires. Would you explain further?

G: Celibacy is helpful to a person keen on making rapid progress on the spiritual path. Breaking celibacy is like spending. When you have some savings in the bank, then you can spend a little. When certain chakras are opening, celibacy is very helpful. However, that does not mean that if you cannot observe celibacy you cannot do sadhana. The second rate path is to earn first and then spend. The third is to just spend and go bankrupt. It is up to you to choose.

D: Is the energy loss during sexual intercourse the same for men and for women, and is the loss in the semen or in the orgasm itself?

G: The loss of energy is the same for both men and women as the orgasm is the loss.

D: Is it really possible for a householder to achieve liberation?

G: Who is not a householder in this world? Who has come into the world without parents or a family? Liberation is for everyone.

D: Even married and working people?

G: Yes, but with one difference. When you eat, you eat, and when you go to the toilet, you go to the toilet. You usually don't try to do both at the same time. Liberation is like eating. Worldly pleasures are like going to the toilet.

Many great saints have been householders. If you go to the jungle to attain realization but your mind is back home with your family and your affairs, your mind will drag you away from your goal. Whatever your style of life, the important thing is the detachment of the mind. Through meditation you will get help. Do what is required in the world and then come back and meditate. God and the guru will give continual help.

D: On one side, a yearning for God is good, but on the other it pulls thoughts and desires into my head and disquiets my mind. I want to have a calm, quiet mind and the yearning disrupts that.

G: The basic difference between God and jivas, individual souls, is that the latter are tied down and dependent whereas God is free and independent. Jivas are many, while God is one. Jivas are bound by Maya, by illusion, whereas God is truth, the ultimate reality. God has no diseases but humans do, so we have to take medicines. Meditation and chanting are such medicines. Once the mind becomes quiet, they are no longer needed. When the mind is not quiet, we must try for quiet. When it has become quiet, it has merged with God. The difference between us as we are now and God is that God is quiet while we are not.

When the universe was created, things divided into opposite qualities which keep it in a rough kind of balance. If everyone becomes a saint, the world will not go on. If everyone becomes a householder, even then the world will not go on. Happiness and unhappiness, good and evil, good people and bad people, these opposite qualities of things are always there. Demons and deities, poison and nectar, day and night, deserts and fertile lands, holy places and unholy places, the whole universe has these two aspects. Saints and rishis have shown the path we must follow to get liberated from all that.

Just as you must work to get a college degree, you must also work to attain peace of mind. People do not mind working 10 years to get a Ph.D., yet on the spiritual path they often get impatient if they do not get peace within a day or two. The college degree is of no use to us after

the present life ends, but the spiritual progress we attain in this life remains with us always. Through this work our minds grow strong, so
have patience and keep working.

D: In school we can measure increments of success, but it's difficult to
measure success in meditation.

G: Just as when we eat, little by little we feel satisfied, and finally automatically we know we are full, so when we develop spiritually, we will know
it. When we are eating we do not put our hands in our stomachs to see
how far the food has reached.

D: Is there a process for developing healing power through meditation?

G: Once you learn to become one-pointed, you will not only have healing
power but also other capacities. Spiritual progress will also lead to creativity in the arts, etc. It brings forth all the talents and powers you may
try for.

D: Is it all right to send Shakti to people mentally if you know they
need help?

G: You should be very careful in doing that. For example, if that person
wants to go out and murder someone but has a fever which is prevent-
ing him from doing it, by sending him your energy you can cause him
to get well and commit the murder. You have to be very careful.

D: Can we use our powers to help other people?

G: Not until you have enough power of your own. If I want to give someone a thousand dollars, I can do so only if I have already saved the money.

D: We made a commitment to keep the healing techniques you taught us
here (at the *Vajra Panjar* retreat) a secret, but can we tell a husband or
wife who is not here?

G: Until you have attained the power, you should keep it a secret—even from a husband or wife. If you sow a seed, you keep it covered until it sprouts. If you keep it open it will die. In any yogic technique, if you do not keep it a secret, you might not attain the power. Until you are given permission to use it for healing, you must keep it a secret.

In India there was a shepherd who had a lot of goats and sheep that he kept in the jungle. Their little huts in the village did not have room for the animals, but whenever a goat or sheep gave birth to a little one they would bring it home. Wolves would eat them if left in the jungle. Once, a goat gave birth to a kid-goat and the shepherd was bringing it back home. On the way he met six thieves. All six started thinking how they could get the kid-goat from him. The shepherd's house was about five or six miles from there. One of the six thieves came to the shepherd and asked him what he was carrying.

The shepherd said, "This is a kid-goat." The thief said, "No, this is a baby wolf," and the thief went away.

Half a mile farther along, another thief came by and also asked him what he was carrying. The shepherd answered that it was a kid-goat. That thief also said, "No, this is a baby wolf." The shepherd said, "Don't tell me that. I just saw it being born from a goat. There is no chance of a mistake." Then he met the third thief who asked the same thing and to whom he gave the same answer. The third thief said the same thing; "This is a baby wolf. Because it is so dark in the jungle maybe you could not see whether it was a goat or a wolf giving birth."

The shepherd began having doubts. He wondered if it really was a wolf. After another half mile the fourth thief came by. The same conversation took place. He said, "You are really a fool. The mother wolf must be close." The shepherd's doubts became stronger and he thought he had made a mistake. Maybe it really was a wolf. The fifth thief came by and said the same thing. The faith that the shepherd had that it really was a kid-goat was completely shaken. He thought to himself, "All five of these people have told me that this is a baby wolf. Why should they lie?"

Then came the last thief. The same conversation took place. This one was the most emphatic. "Throw the baby wolf here before the mother wolf comes and eats you up!" he said. The shepherd threw down the kid-goat and the thief picked him up.

So, a lot of spiritual practices are fruitful but with doubts and dilemmas, the fruit is lost. While you are working on sadhana, do not discuss it, keep it a secret. To attain the fruit of yoga, japa, austerities, mantras and sadhana, it is advised that you keep them a secret until you attain the fruit. If the person with whom you talk is equally involved in it, it is all right to discuss it. But if you are faced with a person who has doubts, it is better to keep it to yourself. Some people have the habit of discussing new things with a lot of other people. God knows your efforts and wishes. You are not going to gain anything by discussing it with other people. It is between you and God.

Another aspect of this is if a person starts to think that they are better than another person. This attitude can get in the way of his progress and then the downfall would begin. The yogis who have discovered the subtle techniques also understand human limitations very well. They know that when the ego gets in the way, various limitations start that can get in the way of attainment. Desires, greed, anger, jealousy, etc. can cause several kinds of physical and mental diseases. By discussing these things before you are perfected, it is likely that your desire to show off will increase so much that you cannot attain and you will fall.

D: Some healers seem more effective in healing a specific ailment, while others have more success with another specific ailment. Why?

G: If there is a fire in one corner of a house, you should put the water directly on it. If you put the water on some other part, the fire will not be put out and the part you put water on may be damaged. So you must know where the disease is, what it is, and why it is there. When you know this accurately, there will be 100% success in the healing. Healing is a science. It is like adding two and two if you understand the "what, where and why" of the illness. After you do the healing treatment, prana-Shakti has to do its work. If you direct the healing energy to the wrong place, it will forcefully break its way through. The healing energy will follow the thought you send with it. If you don't understand the disease and send the energy to the wrong place, you may damage that healthy part. The fact that you can help in certain kinds of illnesses but not in others shows that you do not understand the causes. Shakti is infallible. It will work if you understand how to use it correctly.

D: I have found that I can heal others but I cannot heal my own pain. Why not?

G: When a doctor is sick, he does not treat himself. He cannot himself figure out how he should be treated. When one is sick, one's mental powers are weakened and one cannot heal oneself. The same is true in your case. You do not have enough self-confidence.

D: Can you heal an addiction problem?

G: There are many cases where, after Shaktipat, a disciple gives up smoking on his own, without persuasion or effort.

D: I understand that all diseases originate on the subtle level and that healing is permanent only when the consciousness is changed. Otherwise, they recur in a different form.

G: If a plant seems to be dying and you want to revive it, you have to water the roots. It does no good to water the stem and leaves. Any technique works perfectly only if it can affect all three bodies: the physical, the subtle, and the causal. That is why it is important to awaken the Kundalini. Once awakened, it affects all three levels and the changes it makes are permanent. Also, there are specific kriyas that can be used for various purposes, a specific technique for stomach problems and so forth. Also, there are techniques by which, just as we can travel great distances in a dream, a yogi can take out his subtle body and travel anywhere. It is easy to talk about these techniques but they are difficult to master. Only with the guidance of a perfected guru can one attain them. Yogis have found keys to open many locks. The doors are closed to us and the locks are very big, but if you can get the keys from the yogis, they are easy to open.

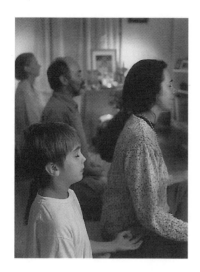

Experiences Along The Path

THE FOLLOWING ARE EXCERPTS from some of the many letters that disciples have sent to me describing their own experiences. They include subjective experiences in meditation, changes in personality and lifestyle, and the spontaneous healing of various illnesses. I think they will be helpful to people on this path so that they can see that experiences that may come to them are not extraordinary or harmful and so that they will not be afraid.

However, it should be emphasized that these experiences describe side effects only. The main thrust of the process of the awakening of the Kundalini is the realization of the true nature of the Self, the ultimate union of jiva and God which brings a complete and permanent end to the suffering of the limited and Maya-bound form of existence. We are not doctors of the body but physicians of the spirit. The healing that sometimes occurs is a side benefit, an added bonus if you will, of the early stages of the process.

Not everyone has such experiences as these. Those that do, have need of them. Those that do not, have no such need. Each person is different and the Shakti works with the situation She finds, doing just what is necessary in each case. These kriyas occur for the purification of the subtle and physical bodies. Even if they become very severe, there is no cause for fear since they will pass when the purification is completed. One should just be patient.

I am writing to tell you of some experiences I've had recently. Last Friday I had taken the children to Shackleford Creek to swim. I was walking out into the water when I saw Christ rising out of the water with his hand in a blessing. I closed my eyes so I could see him better and asked him why he should appear to me since I am so worldly. He told me I was pure in heart. His presence made me full of joy and peace. He was there for awhile, then slowly disappeared, but the happiness I felt with him returns now as I am writing.

About a week before that I was lying down in the heat of the afternoon and you appeared and answered some of my questions. Then a girl about 10 years old, very slender, with a bracelet on each wrist, came and put her arms around my neck. That made me deeply happy. I thought she was the spirit of the child that is growing within me now.

I am writing to ask you if these experiences are real. I tend to trust them all implicitly, and yet I don't trust my own ego and its ability to make things up to please itself.

One night last week I was very tired and wanted to lie down when T. broke a gallon jar of milk in the refrigerator. I got up to help clean up and suddenly you were standing right next to me calmly smiling. I felt a new burst of energy and cheerfulness and T. and I cleaned up the mess easily.

One time recently our cow got out in the middle of the night. When I discovered it the next morning I was afraid she might be miles away, and we might not be able to find her, or else she might have gotten into the alfalfa fields nearby and eaten herself sick. I prayed to you, Gurudev, to help me find her and then I started walking. I walked right to where she was eating grass in the neighbor's yard! T. tracked her and said she did walk miles, but by your grace, Gurudev, when I needed to find her she was not far away.

In so many ways, Gurudev, you are with me. When I forget, I need only to pray and you come. All of us disciples are so blessed and indebted to you. There is no way to repay the love of a true guru. There is no love like the love that comes from a true guru. Gurudev, I could keep writing forever, for though you are like God to me, you are also my Best Friend. But this must be enough for now.

I am very grateful for all your blessings.

Monday, May 2, 1977

I went to the ashram in Scott's Valley because my friend said that a guru there had changed her life. I was very curious, hopeful, but doubtful... I was afraid to be transformed; yet somehow hoped His presence would affect me... I believed myself too headstrong and egotistical to give myself up to a guru, but I wanted to see it happen. I wanted to feel the call to initiation so my life might have more meaning... His chanting was interesting and peaceful. I felt a rush of energy as he came before me, walking through the audience. In the silence that followed I went into meditation, but was too aware of his presence and the sounds of others to go deeply into it. I decided to go again the following night to see if the experience would be any different.

Tuesday, May 3, 1977

During meditation I tested this guru. I prayed, "If you are really my true guru, I want a sign. I would like to experience a kriya." Immediately I found myself sobbing. My breath cut in my throat in short, quick gasps for a few seconds, all involuntarily. Yet this was not enough to convince me. I thought it was caused by autosuggestion. I prayed again, "If you are my guru, I want another sign. I want you to come and touch me on my head." I hardly thought it possible that he would leave his chair in front of the room to touch me. But within a few moments I heard a noise and felt him removing my glasses. Then he touched me on my head. I then went into deep meditation, and when I awoke I felt joyful and thankful.

After meditation I approached the guru and tried to thank him for my experiences, but I was so overcome with feelings of joy and awe that words were difficult to find. Yet I did manage to express to him my fear of initiation. He asked why, and I said, "because of my Catholic mother, because my husband would object, and because it's nothing I planned to do this week." However, without committing myself, I asked for information on Shaktipat.

Wednesday, May 4, 1977

I had difficulty meditating tonight and silently asked for help. Guruji came to me and touched my head. Immediately my spine straightened out, my head tilted back, and my nasal passages cleared so I breathed better. Before I went into meditation, during deep breathing, my breath again choked into sobs, my jaw dropped open, and my tongue rolled back in my throat. I then had a good meditation. Afterwards Guruji told the other disciples how I had examined him. Then he turned to me where I knelt and asked, "Now what do you want?" I replied, "I want initiation." During Shaktipat, I felt a wave of energy moving up from my knees and fingers to my head. Earlier I had asked for one more bit of evidence that these experiences were real. I silently prayed that I might somehow know what Indian name Guruji would give me. And I knew it would be impossible for me to guess, since I knew no Indian names. But after class one of my students came to speak with me about a paper she had written on Sufism, and she told me that the name she was given at her own initiation was "Moti." After Shaktipat, Guruji named me Moti.

Friday, May 6, 1977

Guruji's instructions were to put God and good works before any other work, to lead a regular life, and to meditate daily, all of which I plan to do. I am becoming devoted. I have the strong urge to leave my life and follow the spiritual path uniquely.

As Guruji passed me during meditation, I felt a strong vibration move up from my feet to my hands which tingled. I fell asleep and dreamed that my body was beginning to float out of the bed. A pull down door had begun to open above the closet in my room, and in fear I thought it significant. At this point I asked for help, saying, "O Gurudev, please stop my kriya." The first time I said it, I found myself rising from the dream to another, more conscious level. The second time I said it, I realized I had been dreaming, and the third time, I became fully awake.

Friday, May 20

Today I went into meditation more quickly. A few times I went into rapid automatic breathing. Then my breathing grew so heavy and forceful that my whole body shook from each breath from deep in my diaphragm. Before long I was sobbing, then crying out loud, my mouth open and twisted in a grotesque frown. This cry then diminished into sobs. Then my meditation quickly deepened. My eyes nearly crossed and I felt I was focusing deeply into my own skull. My body began to relax into almost a state of numbness. As all this happened, I was feeling very close to Guruji. I felt that he was with me, protecting and guiding my meditation. At one point, I had a fleeting vision of a seated man, a half-naked Yogi raising a bit of cloth, or some semi-circular object, to his forehead. His face reminded me of pictures of Babaji I had seen. I remained awake during this meditation although it was deep.

At one point, I had slight visions of light traceries of curtains in the shape, perhaps, of a dome, enfolding me as they unfolded a vision of what appeared to be human figures above me. I rose to consciousness, but resumed my mantra and again went into a deeper meditative place that was blank and peaceful, although I did not go out. Suddenly I rose to full consciousness, and my eyes opened. I felt very devotional towards Guruji. I am encouraged that I am making some progress.

ॐ ॐ ॐ

After practicing Zen for some seven years, I met Dhyanyogi Madhusudandasji quite by accident in November of 1976, shortly after he arrived in the United States.

I had just completed giving a lecture when a man told me that a very powerful master of Kundalini Yoga was at the East-West Center a few blocks away. I was not interested. However, after eating a leisurely lunch and not having anything in particular to do that Sunday afternoon, I wandered over to the East West Center to take a look at this fellow.

When I arrived, Guruji was not in the hall. Only a few people were chanting bhajans. I sat down in a correct Zen, "full lotus" posture and proceeded to wait. People began filling up the room and chanting. It felt very peaceful.

After about 45 minutes, Guruji returned from his lunch. He appeared to be a small man, wearing a towel and a ski-cap on his head, who did not speak much in English. He sat down and soon began to chant Sanskrit mantras. My meditation instantly deepened to a state of clear silence inside with the mantras in very sharp focus, like the kind of meditation state one usually achieves on the third or fourth day of an intensive meditation retreat.

Guruji finished his Mantrochar and sat silently for another 20 minutes or so. Then the group sang an Arati, Guruji got up, smiled, said "Everyone be happy," and left.

Suddenly I noticed that I was still sitting in full lotus, although more than two hours had passed, and that my body as well as my mind felt calm and peaceful. Up to that time, I could only maintain such a posture for about half an hour before my legs became very painful.

I came back the next day and received Shaktipat the following week. After that, my meditations went through about a year of heavy breathing and body jerking kriyas. These were subjectively very interesting and I became more aware of energy states and levels within my body. As these kriyas subsided, my meditations took on once again that deep, crystal clear quality of the first meditation with Guruji and have continued that way since.

Although formally they are quite different (closed eyes and relaxed body instead of open eyes and upright body, surrendering to movements of the body instead of holding it still), Dhyanyoga meditation is not different from good Zen meditation. At least, once the Shakti gets its pathways open and the gross kriyas subside, the subjective quality of the two is not different. The chatter of the discursive mind drops away. Feeling states become detached and somewhat distant, almost as if they belonged to someone else. When the eyes are shut, the visual world becomes a velvety blackness filled with tiny points of light and the sound world seems boundless. Images spring up now and again, only to dissolve and float away like small summer clouds, but mostly there is the blackness and the little points of light. When the eyes open and for some time afterwards, the world of forms seems no more than the images that come out of the imagination, constructions the mind measures out of the chaos of sense impressions.

As these experiences grow out of the meditations and color more and more of my everyday life, the world becomes far less serious and my attitude toward it far more open and playful. Without any thought of renunciation or of giving up anything, many outworn old habits just drop away by themselves. As one quits trying to hold onto anything, the sense of freedom and the ability to act efficiently grow.

All of these processes had already begun in my Zen practice. What my meeting Guruji did was to give them a sudden and massive acceleration.

Further, I have learned that whether one bows before the Buddha or chants "Ram" is unimportant. Whether one describes the process as the opening up of the mind or the raising of the Kundalini is only a matter of using language that the hearer can respond to. That the ignorant identification of one's self with this small mind and body and this one life all drops away, so that one can directly know what you and I really are—that is what is important. Dhyanyoga is a powerful tool to aid that awakening.

Guruji has the ability to aid people along this path and he uses it freely, like the rain that falls everywhere and benefits everything that can respond to it. His presence in America is a gift and a blessing to us all.

This is an incident I had that illustrates the power of a Sankalpa.

I was asked to pick up another disciple at Los Angeles airport shortly after New Year's Day, when holiday traffic was still at maximum levels. The arrival time was to be 3:00 on a United Airlines flight from Hawaii. I was at the terminal gate 15 minutes before the plane was scheduled to arrive. Amazingly enough, the 747 was right on time. I watched for the disciple that I was to meet (I will call her Joy.) After watching more than 300 people with beautiful flowers and nice tans get off the plane, and she wasn't one of them, I began to worry a little bit. Just when the last people were trailing out of the gate, I heard my name called on the loud speaker. I went to the phone and the message was that Joy would not be coming until 6:10. That was all, no flight number, no indication of the airline, or even where the message had come from. I assumed at that point that it would be a United Airlines flight since she was supposed to come on United and since I got the message in the United terminal. The only airplane coming in at that time was from San Francisco, to arrive at 6:09. I thought that must be the correct flight, and that she must have somehow gone to San Francisco and then connected down to Los Angeles.

I spent the next two hours wandering around various parts of the airport, watching people, saying malas, and hoping that it was not all in vain. In the waiting I had gotten a little confused as to exactly where the plane would arrive. By the time the plane was supposed to get there I was waiting in the wrong place, and had to race to the other gate some distance away. I got there just as the passengers were getting off, but again Joy was not one of them. I thought that I might have missed her and that she might be at the baggage area. I went down to the baggage area, but there were two different places that the baggage came to, so I spent the next half an hour running between the two. I thought that if I had missed her, she would surely be out on the street waiting for a ride or looking for me. I looked all around but just couldn't find her. I also had her paged over the loud speaker, but to no avail. At that point, after being in the airport hysteria for almost four hours, I was getting just a little tired of it all and wanted to leave. As a last resort I called the house where Guruji was staying to see it they had heard any news of her. They hadn't. After the phone call I decided that I needed some extra help, so I did a sankalpa to Guruji to help me find Joy or to find out somehow that she wasn't at the airport. Then, in a last ditch effort, I decided to walk over to the P.S.A. terminal and see if a flight had come in at 6:10.

All this time I was assuming that she had come to San Francisco and from there was flying to Los Angeles. As I was walking into the P.S.A. terminal (also shared by Continental), lo and behold who should be walking just a few paces ahead of me but the missing Joy! It turned out that she had just done a Sankalpa to find me. The problem was that she had taken a Continental flight from Hawaii but I had not gotten that part of the message. And so you can see how the power of a Sankalpa works. After I related this story to Guruji, he told me that it was right to use the Sankalpa in this way, but that it should be used only in the time of great need, or for spiritual work.

∾ ∾ ∾

While he was at my house, I mentioned to Guruji that my expenses far exceeded my income and that I was in need of additional sources of income. "Don't worry," said Guruji. "You will have plenty of money. You will see."

Results were not long in coming. Within a few days after asking Guruji's help, I received a gift of $1,000 worth of stock from my father. He stipulated that I shouldn't spend it, but there it is for an emergency fund if I should need it. About a week after that, the State Supreme Court ruled that the wage freezes imposed because of the passage of Proposition 13 were illegal and that wage increases contracted for previously would have to be granted. For me, this will mean a lump sum payment of an amount approximately equal to that needed for my son's college housing payment at just about the time it is due, as well as an increase in income of $40.00 per month. Benefits began to come to others in the house as well. First of all, the young man living with us sold his old car for $150.00, enough to pay a bill which he was worried about. Another young man, who visited while Guruji was there, suddenly decided to join the Navy, passed his Navy exam with a score of 98%.

For a long time I have been concerned about my 20-year old son's activities and companions. I wished there would be some way he could leave Los Angeles. However, he seemed so deeply involved and attached that it didn't seem possible that he would leave. After asking for Guruji's help I found myself able to tell him that I wanted him to move out. To my surprise, he not only agreed to move out, but he is making enthusiastic plans for a long trip.

All of these blessings are from resources that have been available to me and to the others involved all along, but for some reason, because of karma or because of lack of knowledge of how to open the treasure chest, they were all being withheld. Guruji knows how to turn the key that opens the treasure chest, and once his help is given, the blessings begin to flow. My gratitude and devotion increase daily as I see Guruji's subtle influence at work transforming my life and the lives of my family members. Jai Gurudev!

I had this experience while visiting Los Angeles. My wife, my 18-month old daughter and I had gone to Guruji's birthday retreat and then stayed over to visit our families and to be with Guruji during the two-week meditation program he was giving there. One day we were out working to earn a little extra money, and then had done some shopping. It was soon a lot later than we thought. We both wanted to go to meditation that night, but for a number of reasons it looked like we could not. First of all, we were not exactly sure where we were. Secondly, having no car, we would have to take the bus, but we didn't have any idea how to find our way around by bus. We also had the problem of the baby because we could not take her to the meditation, yet did not have time to take her to my parents and get back in time for the meditation. So we were wondering what to do as we were standing at the bus stop. One bus came by, but because of what it said on the front, we didn't think it was the right one. Then I made a Sankalpa to Guruji for help. We certainly needed it then. The next bus didn't have any markings on it at all. Not knowing what to do we got on the bus to ask for directions, but before we could ask, the doors closed and away we went.

While we were trying to find out from the driver where we were going, a voice called out my name. It turned out to be a friend that I used to go to school with many years ago, and whom I hadn't seen for a long time. It happened that my friend took us to his house that was not far away. He was more than glad to baby-sit our daughter since he also had a young child. We had plenty of time to make it to the meditation. In meeting our old friends and sharing our experiences of being with Guruji, they also came to the meditation programs later that week.

∾ ∾ ∾

During Shaktipat, at one point I heard church bells ringing. These bells had a beautiful tone and were very clear and sounded nearby. I thought they were ringing the church bells in the village. It was only afterwards that the others told me no church bells were rung during that period of time. Even more incredible, the next evening as I was saying the mantra, the church bells again sounded. I was not in meditation as I had only said the mantra a few times. The church bells were further off in the distance but just as clear and lovely. Along with the church bells, I smelled the fragrance of roses even though there were no roses nearby. Since then I have experienced the smell of roses many times, sometimes during meditation, but more often than not while I am going about my daily chores.

During meditation, the most frequent experiences that have occurred have been trembling in the legs and face (these occur almost every time I meditate). I have also had floating sensations, feelings of my body stretching and contracting. I heard sounds like gun shots in the distance and sounds of rushing waters. I have felt tingling, and currents rushing through my body, heat (especially on top of my head), feelings as if the breath has stopped (during these periods the currents are felt most strongly), and a very strong sensation of pulling between the eyes. At these times, my eyes feel squeezed shut. The first time I experienced this sensation, nothing new happened during meditation, but after I had stopped meditating, I closed my eyes and saw a brilliant white light that turned to a bright red. This was the first time I had seen a colored light. Even during Shaktipat the lights I saw weren't colored. Since then I have seen a blue light. It was a bright cerulean blue. I was very fond of this color when I was painting landscapes and used it frequently in the sky. The same evening I saw the red light, I was preparing for bed and had just turned on the light, when I noticed what appeared to be heat lightning flashing outside the window across the room. I assumed we would be getting a storm, when it suddenly occurred to me that the weather had been cool and clear, not hot and humid as it is when lightning occurs; also the drapes were pulled, so I could not have seen the lightning anyway. At this point, I must admit I got scared and turned away. I then tried to collect myself, as I knew that I shouldn't be afraid, and finally gathered enough courage to look again. This time I saw a glow of light quite large that is very difficult to describe, except that I have never seen such a light before. It seemed to be a transparent ball of light in the center, which was surrounded by a glowing halo. This is a very inadequate description, but it's as close as I can come. As I looked, it appeared to move towards me. This really frightened me and I turned away again and didn't look back. Finally I fell asleep. One thing I am very sure of is that I was not asleep or dreaming when this occurred. In fact, I had been standing by my bed, very alert and wondering how I would be able to fall asleep when the light flashed at the window. Later I asked people if there had been a storm that night, and there had not. I am convinced this was a divine occurrence. This is the first time that such a miraculous thing has taken place in my life, as I am not given to psychic experiences. I could not believe that I was having these experiences, wide-awake, and not in a dream or in meditation. I am forever grateful to you for allowing me to experience the divine power of God, and only regret that I was not calm enough to contemplate the event longer. However, in general I experience an inner peace I have not known in my life before and all of my physical ailments have vanished. I am sure my hypoglycemia is over, as I have much energy; also, other physical problems such as digestive troubles, a pain in my shoulder and a chronic bladder infection have gone. In general my health is better than it has been in years.

The experiences that one gets at the time of Shaktipat and after during the practice of regular meditation, are mostly subjective and spiritual, and hence difficult to fully describe in words. However, I will try to express whatever I observed and gained at the time of my initiation and during my sadhana period.

I sat with closed eyes, and Gurudev touched me on my forehead between the eyebrows. I felt something like mild electric current flowing in my forehead and scalp, which spread all over the body. It gave me a thrilling sensation. I experienced incredible joy from within. I lost all sense of my physical body and the surroundings. Then I saw a huge sphere of light. It was extremely bright but still not dazzling since it was cool and soothing. Later on, I saw different designs in wonderful colors. My mind became steady and concentrated, immersed in joy never known before. I was totally unaware of space and time. When Gurudev awakened me by a gentle touch on the forehead, I immediately asked him "Why was I awakened? I was totally immersed in joy." Gurudev sweetly explained to me, "One hour has passed. Today is the first day of meditation. You should not sit longer."

This spiritual experience made a deep impression on me. I was changed. While returning home, I felt that my body had become light and fresh. Some new energy had filled every part of my body. I felt at least 25 years younger. It reminded me of my student age. My gait had suddenly changed. It became fast with longer, quicker steps and without any strain. Mentally I felt very calm, happy and contented. I realized that today, by the grace of my Gurudev, I attained something very precious.

Thereafter I could go to Gurudev for meditation only for five days. Every time I had wonderful experiences. On the 6th day, I had to leave for my native town. So I took leave of my Gurudev. He blessed me and told me, "Now your Kundalini is awakened, and wherever you go, you will get the same type of meditation. You have to continue regular practice of meditation. This Divine Power will look after you like a mother, will help in your spiritual progress and will take you to your supreme goal." In my native place, I continued my meditation program regularly for one hour in the morning and one hour in the evening. I used to get fairly good concentration with some divine visions. I was convinced that by the grace of my Gurudev I had a glimpse of my cherished goal. He has not only shown me the path to the goal, but he has held my hand and is leading me to it.

As my practice of meditation continued, I started to experience prana Shakti working in different parts of my body. Sometimes I felt the sensation of an insect crawling along my spine. Occasionally I used to have a sensation of heat on some part of the body, or even the whole body, during meditation. For some days I could feel the pulsation in different parts of my body, especially over the neck and scalp, and I could even hear my heartbeats and count them. Sometimes my heart used to beat fast, and sometimes slow. All these experiences gave me great pleasure and peace during my meditation. Later on, activities of prana Shakti were experienced not only during meditation, but during all 24 hours in the form of some current flowing along the nerves in different parts of my body, especially the forehead and scalp. Many times I would experience involuntary movements of my body, and even tremors in some muscles. Sometimes my body involuntarily assumed different yogic poses. On other occasions I used to have various involuntary pranayama, breathing exercises. Although all these experiences gave me extra pleasure and peace of mind, I doubted whether I was on the correct path. So I wrote to Gurudev about these. He immediately replied to me in a sweet way. He explained, "When the Kundalini Shakti is awakened by Shaktipat, She becomes active and starts purification of the body and the mind. Your experiences are due to the activities of prana Shakti —the power of the Kundalini Shakti. Forceful flow of prana in the nerves to remove the impurities in physical or subtle forms give rise to sensations of heat, involuntary movements, yogic poses, pranayama and other experiences. When impurities are removed, one gets peaceful meditation."

As I carried on my regular practice of meditation, I experienced some of the signs of vital centers of chakras being pierced by the Kundalini Shakti, which were described and explained to me by Gurudev in those days in his letters. One night, about eight months after my Shaktipat, I had a very unique experience during meditation. It was June 1963. As usual, I sat for meditation at about 10:30 p.m. In the beginning I had a fair amount of concentration, but all of a sudden I felt a cool breeze blowing and my body getting cold. I almost lost consciousness. I felt, I am leaving my body. I saw a small golden ball leaving my body. I was in that ball. The ball was slowly soaring up higher and higher in the sky. I saw my body lying still on the floor. But I was experiencing indescribable bliss. I do not know how long I remained in that stage. When I awoke it was 12 p.m. This extraordinary, thrilling experience had given extra freshness to my body and extra peace and happiness to my mind. I could not understand what it was due to. After about 15 days, when Gurudev arrived in Bombay, I described my experiences to Him. He was glad to hear it and explained to me that I was very fortunate. It was a rare experience. He told me that I had reached the Sahasrara, i.e., my Kundalini Shakti had pierced all the chakras and reached the top. He was satisfied that I had progressed well.

Afterwards Gurudev stayed with us for two months. Practicing meditation in his vicinity, my family and I made very quick progress, with a lot of spiritual experiences.

ॐ ॐ ॐ

I went to see the ashram in Yreka last weekend. We all felt your presence at the meeting, guiding us. I saw the ashram land in a meditation last December. Here is what I wrote in my diary:

12/10/77

Last night in meditation, I saw some land and a house. Tonight I saw the same land and house. There were rolling hills, trees on both sides, and a small pond. I heard Guruji say, "The people involved will know in their hearts that this is the right place because we have all already seen it, so we will recognize it." Guruji then said that the land will not have to be subdivided—money will come.

I had forgotten about seeing the land until I walked toward the back of the ashram and stood in the same place I had been in my meditation. I looked down the same rolling hills with trees on both sides. I felt such awe for you and God.

I have been praying to you and Shiva for guidance. Thursday night I felt you both in my room—the energy so intense I couldn't sleep. I felt such love and gratitude to you for coming. I had been feeling confused and lonely. I strongly felt you both telling me to go to the ashram now.

This morning, I woke up in a deep meditation. This happens a lot now. I knew I had to get up but I was with you, Guruji, and I didn't want to leave.

Lately I am much at ease. I have no more fears. I can begin meditating without difficulty, and my meditations seem longer and deeper. My hands continue to form mudras, and now my teeth have begun chattering for short periods of time. Mostly my mind is blank during meditation. I hear nothing, see nothing, and yet feel clear and aware, not asleep. And I feel calm and refreshed afterwards. There have been a few days when I have felt as though I were meditating all day. I would teach my classes and hold conferences with my students, but I would feel less a part of these outer activities than of my participation in some inner world. This is hard to explain, but I am trying to thank you for your help, for how effortless life is becoming. Without trying so hard, without worrying, my work is getting done. My mind has lost many of its questions and doubts, although it invents new ones from time to time. I pray always to be completely surrendered, devoted, faithful.

More and more I feel you with me and have faith you are with me. The greatest gift I've received this lifetime is your grace and my devotion to you. I love you, my dear Guruji, and will serve you in any way I can. Please keep my heart open.

All my life, I have been very allergic to poison oak that would give me a miserable rash that would last for months. I now have a job in an orchard where I am constantly exposed to the plant. The only thing that medical doctors have done was to prescribe a strong antibiotic that made me very susceptible to any diseases I might be exposed to and, as I was also working in a hospital at the time, that was very dangerous.

Gurudev gave me a mantra to say if I became infected with poison oak. I faithfully followed his instructions, and each time the rash would dry up and go away in a few days.

∾ ∾ ∾

[A medical doctor in Bombay]

If the aspirant is thin and lean, he or she will gain weight and become normal. There was a young girl of 20 who was thin and underweight. After Shaktipat she gained 10 pounds in 15 days with her usual diet.

If the aspirant is obese and overweight, he or she will lose weight until it comes to a normal level without dieting. This is my personal experience. At the time of my Shaktipat I was overweight by about 15 pounds. Even with restricted dieting, I could not reduce it. But after initiation and regular practice of meditation, I lost my 15 pounds within the first three months, even with a normal diet. My second son, who was 16 at the time of his Shaktipat, was slightly overweight. He lost his extra weight, and his body became quite proportionate with practice of meditation. There are many such cases observed by us.

Similarly, we have observed many physical diseases, medical or surgical, minor or major, acute or chronic, being cured by Kundalini Shakti when She is awakened by the grace of our Gurudev. Any organ of the body gets diseased due to partial or total loss of life energy in the cells of that organ, due to infection, trauma, poisoning, etc. The Kundalini, when awakened by Shaktipat, supplies fresh life energy, or prana Shakti, to the cells of that organ, during regular practice of meditation, and the part regains complete health. I have seen cases of sciatica, peptic ulcer, hypertension, heart trouble, insomnia, soft ankylosis, frozen joints, etc., totally cured after Shaktipat and regular practice of meditation. Acute ailments and joint sprains were instantly cured by the action of prana Shakti during meditation.

∾ ∾ ∾

135

One aspirant who was about 60 years old fell from a moving bus and fractured his left humerus. Even after proper and prolonged treatments, his left shoulder joint became stiff with no movement. He carried on like this for many months, but on one fine morning, while he was in meditation, prana Shakti worked. He got involuntary movements of that joint. On awakening from meditation, to his great joy, he found that he could move his left shoulder joint quite freely and absolutely without pain.

Similarly, there was a case of one elderly lady who had also injured her shoulder joint and had the same trouble. Her joint had soft ankylosis and was treated by expert doctors, but it did not improve even with prolonged treatment. Once, while she was in meditation, prana Shakti made her joint move involuntarily. Since then her trouble is gone and she can move that joint quite freely without pain.

There is a third such case of a gentleman about 50 years old who had already been initiated by Gurudev when, because of an injury, he experienced pain and stiffness of one knee joint. He felt very unhappy that he could not bend his knee and sit for meditation in his usual posture with crossed legs. Gurudev advised him not to worry, and to carry on meditation with extended legs. One day a wonderful thing happened: prana Shakti worked during meditation. He had involuntary flexion of his knee joint. On awakening he found that he could bend his knee easily without any pain. He was overwhelmed with joy, prostrated himself before Gurudev, thanked him for his grace and danced in joy.

In Bombay, we had a meditation center about 1 1/2 miles away from my clinic. Gurudev was out of Bombay, but I had made it a rule to visit our center every night after finishing work in my clinic. On the previous day I had badly sprained my right ankle while walking, and I had severe pain with marked swelling over the joint. I could walk only with great difficulty. But on that day somehow I managed to visit the center and sit for meditation. I had deeper concentration that day. To my surprise I experienced continuous activity of prana Shakti over my injured joint, with such a severe heat that I thought sparks might come out of that area. When I awoke

I saw that the swelling and pain had totally disappeared, and I could walk comfortably on the road.

I had a peptic ulcer since July 1961, and it would not respond to ordinary treatment of antacids, anticholenergics, tranquilizers, and a strictly bland diet. Only continuous heavy doses of these drugs with severe restrictions in my diet used to give me some relief from epigastric pain and burning in the chest and stomach. I did not talk to Gurudev about this ailment. At the time of my initiation, I went to Gurudev for only 6 days and there was no change in this trouble. After that, when I went to my native town, to my pleasant surprise, all symptoms of the peptic ulcer suddenly disappeared. I started taking a normal diet without the slightest trouble in my stomach. I thought my peptic ulcer gone forever. This went on for about 3 1/2 months after my initiation, but one morning I was awakened by severe epigastric pain, typical of a peptic ulcer. I was shocked that my peptic ulcer had returned in full form, so I wrote about this to Gurudev. Gurudev kindly replied to me, "Just as you doctors give chloroform and anesthetize the patient, similarly, the Primordial Power, the Kundalini Shakti had taken control of your body for about 100 days and has taken you to the highest stage."

Thereafter, together with regular medical treatment and diet restriction, I carried on with my regular practice of meditation. One day someone told my wife that my chronic peptic ulcer would lead to cancer of the stomach. My wife was frightened on hearing this and got nervous. Immediately she went to Gurudev and prayed to him to have mercy on us and save me. Gurudev at once told her not to worry at all and assured her that "Prana Shakti will work and the peptic ulcer will be healed within 1 1/2 years." To our pleasant surprise, all the symptoms of my peptic ulcer totally disappeared exactly after 1 1/2 years and have never recurred.

The Kundalini, when awakened, starts functioning and supplies fresh life energy, or prana, to every cell of the brain and other organs. Brain cells thereby get rejuvenated. Thus, meditation works as a great tonic to brain and nerves, as a result of which intelligence improves, becoming sharp and subtle. One starts grasping subtle subjects of higher philosophy and spiritualism. Memory improves. Judging capacity improves. One can come to quick decisions, even about difficult problems. Thus meditation proves very helpful even in office work, business, and day to day life. Whatever work one could turn out before in eight hours, he can then dispose of in three hours with great efficiency and less strain.

I have resolved a very deep conflict that has been bothering me for some time.

I have realized what has been tearing my heart in two. I had been thinking that the love I felt so strongly was my love for the Guru—the form. Because of this I experienced intense longing to be with you—also in form. I have had many recent prolonged experiences, both in and out of meditation, of the love and magnificence of God—everywhere. At first this tortured my heart more because I thought of you constantly. I feel your presence all the time. Perhaps it is truer to say that the peace and love and harmony I feel now are the same as being with you. The energy of unbounded love permeates everything.

Guruji, you have shown me the way to experience my own inner self—to realize my own heart, to feel the presence of the inner Guru. To look outside one's own self to find God is only half the truth. Our minds can "believe" that God's love is everywhere, but only our hearts can truly see.

Now I understand the blessings you have given me. The oneness and the overgrowing love inside me are also in you. There is no difference. *So Ham* — I AM THAT... Everywhere... Forever...

There are so many things in my heart to tell you. Mostly I want to talk to you about how I should earn my living. I pray for guidance. It is clear to me now that I want my life to be one of devotion and service to God. The only reason for income is to keep going. I want to work for God in whatever I do. I want to do whatever God wants me to do so that He can provide for me while I serve Him.

A wonderful example of this came two days ago. My motorcycle was broken, and I could not fix it. The mechanic said it would cost about a hundred dollars to repair it. I hardly had enough to live on. I was in despair. I renewed my devotions. I got my thinking straight that God would provide for me if I but serve Him. I called upon you to help me. I began saying the mantra again to purify myself as I walked the streets.

Just then the art gallery where I have my paintings called me to come down, and they gave me a new, crisp $100 bill! The right person had suddenly come and bought one.

I have been a teacher all my adult life, but now I feel that I am supposed to be doing a different kind of teaching, and to get my income some other way. Next month I will be starting a class at the college here with the idea of using it to bring disciples to you. Besides the regular classes, there is a branch called the University for Man. I am planning to teach people how to work on the emotional distresses in their lives that get in the way of being able to meditate. This is mostly counseling work, and I shall teach what I have taught before. But what is new for me comes from the fact that now you have transformed my life. A good teacher does not teach what he knows; he teaches what he is. And so, I will share my self, my own journey along the path, and will try to help my students become familiar with the ways of meditation you teach.

When I first attended one of your meditations, I could not accept you because it was all too strange, too foreign to my eyes. I will gently lead my Western brothers and sisters past those prejudices and start getting them used to the Eastern ways. I cannot teach meditation, of course. All I can do is help people get ready, and to want to come to you. That is what being a disciple means to me.

I do not enjoy earth-life much any more. Its pleasures have less and less appeal to me. There is so much distress, so much craziness, and so much blindness. I find it very, very hard to live here. I want so very, very much to go "home." I pray to be released from this earthly cycle. But until then, I pray to be allowed to live a gentle life of service to God for the rest of my days. That is the only way I can see life being worth living.

Each brief time that I have been with you has been on a higher plane than before. Each time has created a whirlwind of change and transformation within me. How I hunger to be with you all the time! And yet, I accept working in the world with your guidance, for I deeply believe you are with me always.

∾ ∾ ∾

My meditations are calm now, not stormy like before. The symbols have quieted for now; so have the verses. But I can still feel Kundalini working from within.

Manifestations may not be present within me, but my mind is growing with a new awareness day by day. New ideas can come easily to me, and the old concepts of the past are released easily by me.

I sit sometimes by myself and wonder with amazement at my lifestyle before Guruji came into my life. I feel like Lazarus of the Bible, and have come out of the old tomb, free of the pain and tears. Somehow the old me has died and arisen from the ashes of mental and physical despair.

Guruji has made me realize that all of mankind is born to die in more ways than one. Through meditation I have learned that death is our constant companion; I should have indulged it a little in the past for growth. Before Guruji came I didn't, and began to choke from my old inflexible skin that had toughened with the passionate poisons of stale ideas and wrong ideologies.

Now nothing of the past can satisfy me.

Glossary

[Note on Sanskrit spellings used in this book: As in the original edition, Sanskrit terms have been rendered without diacritical marks and without attempting to discriminate between long and short vowels or the two "sh" sounds. The letter written "c" in the standard orthography has been rendered "ch" here. Otherwise, spellings conform to the standard international system used in the Monier-Williams Dictionary. Thus the spellings here do not give an entirely accurate guide to exact pronunciation. Also many words have become Anglicized to the point of acquiring an English plural "s" (e.g. kriyas) and this usage has been retained here although we are quite well aware that Sanskrit has its own methods for forming dual and plural forms. In doing so, we are simply conforming to the usage that has grown up around these words among practitioners and students of yoga in the United States.]

AJNA

The chakra located between the eyebrows. The name means "towards knowledge. "

AKASHA

Space. One of the eight tattvas (elements). These tattvas compose a living being in the natural world. Space is related to the throat chakra and is the medium for Nada (sound).

ANAHATA

One of the chakras. The heart center.

ANUSTHAN

The carrying out of a spiritual practice, in a specific time and place, for a particular purpose. Literally means 'to stay near' — to the Divine and one's inner Self — uninvolved with the day-to-day world.

APANA-VAYU

One of the five vayu (vital airs). Apana works downward and controls the elimination of all wastes from the body.

ARATI

The ceremony at the close of a meditation when lights are offered to God and Guru, or to his picture and to the images or pictures of deities in the meditation room.

ASHRAM

The place of residence for a spiritual community, or other permanent meeting place for the carrying on of spiritual practices.

ATMA

The Self, one's own self in its absolute aspect; what one really is underneath all of the temporary characteristics one may have (i.e. the soul).

BANDHA

A lock. A technique of closing the body at the anus, the navel, the throat, or all three places, to the flow of prana.

BHAGAVAD GITA

This Scripture is a part of the *Mahabharata* wherein Lord Krishna explains to Arjuna the various forms and practices of yoga and knowledge of the Self.

BHAKTI

Devotion, reverence.

BHAKTI YOGA

A method of union with God through love and devotion to some personalized form of the deity.

BHASTRIKA PRANAYAMA

Breathing like a bellows at a regular and controlled pace, whether slow, medium or fast.

BHUTA SHUDDHI MANTRA

The mantra given by Shri Dhyanyogiji to his disciples after Shaktipat for the protection and purification of their physical, subtle and causal bodies.

BIJA MANTRA

Seed mantra or seed syllable. The basic elements of articulate sound which are inscribed on the petals of the various lotuses at the chakras of the subtle body. They are the seeds from which all mantras are generated and powerful tools for the direction and control of the flow of prana.

BRAHMA

The creative aspect of God, the Demiurge or creator of the universe.

BRAHMAN

The Absolute, ground of all being and becoming.

BRAHMANDA

The "cosmic egg" of Brahma, the created universe.

CAUSAL BODY

One of the three bodies of every living being. It is composed of the habits and patterns (samskaras) formed by actions done in the past and continually evolves with the addition of new karma. The resultant of all one's past volitional actions in this and past lives.

CHAKRA

The centers of activity within the pranic system of the subtle body. There are six such chakras, plus the Sahasrara. All are described in detail in the main text.

DEVA

A deity. A personalized form or aspect of God that personifies certain Divine functions.

DHYANA

In general, meditation. In the technical sense, as used in Raja Yoga, dhyana is that stage in the contemplation of an object when the attention has narrowed to an awareness of the self and the object only.

DHYANYOGA

Union with the Absolute (or God) through meditation.

GANESHA

A form of God, son of Shiva and Shakti. Pictured with the head of an elephant and the body of a man, he personifies the power that bursts through all obstacles and is usually lauded at the beginning of any project. This form gives insight and wisdom.

GOD

A personification of the Absolute. An intermediate form with personality and characteristics through which one may approach the realization of the ultimate, formless Absolute or Brahman.

GRANTHI

Knot. A complex tangle in the pattern of the energy flow that is straightened by the passage of the awakened Kundalini, thus opening to the receipt of knowledge.

GUNAS

The three general qualities into which Prakriti or Nature divided, the general qualities of which all Maya is constituted: Sattva (purity), Rajas (action) and Tamas (darkness).

GURU

A teacher, "Remover of Darkness (ignorance)". Usually implies a spiritual teacher.

GURUDEV

A title of respect meaning, "Oh Teacher, Who Is Like A God to Me."

GURU TATTVA

The Guru principle: the essential nature and Grace of the Guru, which operates independently of the physical form.

HARI

One of the names of God in his Vishnu aspect as maintainer of the universe.

HATHA YOGA

One of the eight limbs of yoga that relies primarily on physical postures (asanas).

HITA NADI

The channel of energy through which one receives energy from the external source, the Sun.

IDA NADI

The secondary nadi, running along the left of the Sushumna, associated with the cooling energy of the Moon.

INDRIYA

A faculty. There are five jnanendriyas, or sense faculties: eye, ear, nose, tongue and skin. There are also five karmendriyas, or action faculties: legs, hands, mouth, genitals and anus.

JAPA

The repetition of a mantra or of one of the names of God.

JIVA

An individual soul. A spark from the fire of God apparently enclosed and separated from God by Maya. Jivatma is another form of the same concept emphasizing the identity of jiva and Atma.

JNANA

Knowledge.

JNANA YOGA

Another of the yogas described in the *Bhagavad Gita*. It depends on knowledge of the actual nature and function of things as a means of liberation.

JNANENDRIYA

The five senses of knowledge: hearing, touch, sight, taste and smell.

KARMA

Action or activity. When used in the sense of one's own karma, it means one's volitional acts in the past, which cause one to be the being one is now. This is not a mystical notion but the simple recognition of the fact that I am, as a person, the sum of what I have done and what I do.

KARMA YOGA

The method of union with God through offering the fruits of all one's actions to God.

KARMENDRIYA

The five organs of action: hands, feet, speech, anus, genitals.

KRISHNA

A name of God. One of the twenty-four avatars of Vishnu. An avatar is an incarnation of Vishnu in various forms, manifested at specific times to restore balance to the universe.

KRIYA

A motion or movement. As used here, the word relates to those involuntary movements made by people in meditation caused by the action of the Kundalini on the body.

KUMBHAKA PRANAYAMA

Retention of breath.

KUNDALINI

The primordial energy. The Shakti coiled and dormant in the Muladhara chakra after it forms the chakra system of the subtle body. Awakened, it retraces its route back to the Sahasrara and creates the conditions for spiritual progress and Self-realization.

LINGAM

A stylized representation of the male generative organ used as a symbol of the creative aspect of God in the form of Shiva.

MAHA

Great or large.

MAHASAMADHI

The final conscious departure from the body of a realized soul.

MAHESHVARA

(Also written Maheshwara, the "v" and "w" being interchangeable in the Romanization of Sanskrit.) The Great Lord, a title of Shiva.

MALA

Garland. A string of 108 beads used for counting repetitions of a mantra.

MANAS CHAKRA

The seat of the human mind at the third eye center.

MANIPURA

The chakra located at the navel.

MANTRA

A sound, or a string of sounds, so organized as to affect the energies of the subtle body in a particular fashion. The sounds may also carry some conceptual meaning but this is entirely secondary.

MANTROCHAR

A specific collection (smaran) of mantras sung by Shri Dhyanyogiji or Shri Anandi Ma at group meditations to help remove blockages at the subtle level and stimulate the movement of the Kundalini to facilitate spiritual progress.

MAYA

Illusion, the world of our daily experience. The term is inclusive of all our perceptions of solid, liquid, radiant and gaseous objects, together with the space that contains them, the mind that experiences them, the intellect that analyses, classifies and thinks about them, and the ego that conceives of itself as something separate from them. Maya is what clouds our perception so that we do not see ourselves in our true state as identical with God.

MAYA SHAKTI

The Shakti, or power of God, of which the universe and all in it is formed.

MULADHARA

The chakra located between the anus and the genitals.

NADA

Sound. A more precise translation would refer not only to the range of audible sound vibrations, but to all the range of vibrations or wave patterns which form substances and energies.

NADI

One of the channels of prana in the subtle body.

NIRGUNA

Without qualities, not composed of a mixture of sattva, rajas and tamas. It is usually applied to that aspect of the Absolute in which it cannot be characterized, described in words or categories, and is beyond all qualities.

NIRVIKALPA SAMADHI

Nir not, *vi* divided into, *kalpa* measures or categories. That state of samadhi where all words and categorization are cut off.

OMKARA

The sound of AUM or OM (almost identical in Sanskrit). Properly pronounced, it contains the full range of all sounds and, being complete, is the sound of God.

PARAMATMA

Param ultimate, extreme; *Atma,* self. The Absolute in its first stage of personification.

PINGALA

The secondary nadi, along the right side of the Sushumna, associated with the heating energy of the Sun.

PRAKRITI

The initial division in the unbroken fabric of the Absolute upon coming into manifestation is the division into Prakriti and Purusha, Nature and Spirit, not-me and me (i.e., what-I-am-not and what-I-am). See *Bhagavad Gita*, Chapter 13, Verses 20 to 24, for a full description.

PRANA

Energy. The "raw material" of Shakti. The distinction between prana and Shakti is like that between energy and power. "Prana Shakti" is a redundancy used for emphasis.

PRANA-VAYU

A wind or current of prana.

PRANAYAMA

The *ayam* (control) of *prana* through regulation of the physical breath, that being the point where the physical and subtle bodies are in closest effective contact. Regulation of the breathing pattern not only affects the energy flow through the physical body, but also controls the emotions and the flow of prana.

PRATYAHARA

The withdrawal of the senses from their objects: introversion of attention.

PURAKA PRANAYAMA

Inhalation. Focus on the incoming, filling breath.

PUJA

Ritual worship of an aspect of the Divine.

PURUSHA

Spirit. See *Prakriti* for a fuller discussion.

RAJAS

The activating quality or *guna*: passion, emotion. Movement, action, acceleration.

RAJA YOGA

The king (*raja*) of yogas. A method of stilling the mind in order to unite with what is beyond the mind.

RAM

Also written *Rama*. Generally, God, but specifically, one of the twenty-four avatars of Vishnu, whose life and deeds are recorded in the *Ramayana*.

RECHAKA PRANAYAMA

Exhalation. Focus on the outgoing, emptying breath.

RISHI

The seers who 'saw' the scriptures. They are not authors for they did not invent nor compose these works, but rather observed them in meditation and wrote them down.

SADGURU

A true or perfected guru.

SADHANA

Spiritual practices going toward Self-realization.

SAHASRARA

The center of pranic activity located at the crown of the head. The thousand-petaled lotus.

SAMADHI

Concentration of thoughts, profound or abstract meditation, contemplation of an object to the point that the contemplator is completely identified with the object contemplated; the eighth and final stage of yoga.

SAMANA-VAYU

The prana that controls digestion and assimilation of materials into body.

SAMSKARA

Patterns of mind or behavior, habits formed as a result of past karma. The personality mask with which the ego usually identifies itself is composed of samskaras.

SANKALPA

A formed intention. The mental determination that a particular action will occur in a certain way. Autosuggestion.

SATTVA

The balancing or harmonizing quality or *guna*: purity, goodness. It balances *rajas*, acceleration, and *tamas*, inertia.

SHAKTI

Power. The active aspect of God. The ability to act. What prana does. For all practical purposes Kundalini and Shakti can be defined in the same way.

SHAKTIPAT

The transfer, *pata*, of Shakti from a perfected guru to his disciple for the purpose of awakening the disciple's Kundalini.

SHIVA

God in His dissolution aspect, and therefore also in his generative aspect. This is because any process of becoming is viewed as a creation or a destruction depending on whether one sees it from the viewpoint of the old that is ceasing to be, or the new which is coming into being. Shiva (literally 'auspicious') points to the process itself with the dual viewpoints discarded.

SO HAM

He, *sah,* and I, *sham,* becomes "So Ham" when the words are put together according to the rules of Sanskrit. The phrase means "He (i.e. God) am I." The correlative phrase is *Hansah,* composed of *aham,* I, and *sah,* He, meaning "I am He." Hansah also means "swan" or "wild goose" and so those high flying, migratory birds become poetic and artistic metaphors for identity of the jiva and God.

SUBTLE BODY

One of the three bodies of each jiva. It is composed of prana, samskaras, feelings, thoughts, emotions, etc.

SUSHUMNA

The central nadi of the subtle body along which the chakras are located and the Kundalini operates. It is closed until the awakened Kundalini forces it open and uses it as a path to return to the Sahasrara.

SVADHISHTHANA

The chakra located between the genitals and the navel.

SVAYAMBHU

Self-existent. A name of Shiva or of Brahman, the uncaused, unoriginated aspect of God.

TAMAS

The quality or *guna* of inertia: slowing or stopping.

TATTVA

A true or real state, a truth or reality, or a true principle. There are various lists of tattvas in various philosophical systems.

TURIYA

The fourth state of Spirit: pure, impersonal Brahman.

UDANA

The prana-vayu connecting the physical and subtle bodies and directing energies towards higher planes. This is located at the throat and helps with swallowing.

UPANISHAD

One of the classes of Indian scriptures. Historically, the Upanishads were written after the Vedas and Brahmanas, and before the development of the six formal philosophical systems and the Puranas.

VAYU

Wind. Here, it usually means prana-vayu or current of energy.

VISHNU

A name for God in His aspect as preserver and maintainer of the universe.

VISHUDDHA

The throat chakra.

VYANA

The prana-vayu controlling circulation and distribution of energies. It separates and disintegrates things as it works throughout the body.

YOGA

Union with God. One who practices yoga is a *yogi* or a *yogini.*

∾∾∾

Index

Recommended Reading

Before beginning intensive meditation practice, all disciples are advised to read two other books written by Shri Dhyanyogiji: *Light on Meditation* and *Message to Disciples*. In addition, the following reading list is suggested:

Raja Yoga by Shri Swami Vivekenanda
— English, Gujarati or Hindi
(Vedanta Press, 1946 Vedanta Place, Hollywood, CA 90068)

Kundalini Yoga, and, *Spiritual Experiences* by Shri Swami Sivananda

Devatma Shakti (Kundalini) Divine Power
by Swami Shri Vishnutirthaji Maharaj — English

1. Shri Sadhan Granthamala Prakashan Samiti, Narayan Kuti, Sanyasashram, Dewas junior, Post Dewas, M.P., India

2. Shri Devendra Vaignyani, Vaignyan Press, Post Rishikesh, Dist: Dehradun, U.P., India

Shaktipat and other books by Swami Shri Vishnutirthaji Maharaj — Gujarati or Hindi

Vartalap by Shri Mataji — Gujarati or Hindi